From Ow
to
Wow!

Five Steps to
Thriving with Pain

Amber Rose Dullea, MA, M.Div

Typeset: Greg Salisbury
Book Cover Design: Marla Thompson
Editor: Kristin Sanders
Portrait Photographer: Rhiannon Griffiths

DISCLAIMER: This book has been created to inform individuals with an interest in taking back control of their own health. It is not intended in any way to replace other professional health care or mental health advice, but to support it. Readers of this publication agree that neither Amber Rose Dullea nor her publisher will be held responsible or liable for damages that may be alleged or resulting, directly, or indirectly, from their use of this publication. All external links are provided as a resource only and are not guaranteed to remain active for any length of time. Neither the publisher nor the author can be held accountable for the information provided by, or actions resulting from accessing these resources. All opinions in this book are those of the author.

Dedication

To those who live with chronic pain and want to take your life back and thrive. And to Rhiannon, my Partner who has been on this journey and who thrives with me every day.

Testimonials

"Unlike books that cover pain management techniques or encourage attitude adjustment, From Ow to Wow! gives readers a full spectrum approach to changing their relationship with pain and taking effective action towards a life worth living. Amber Rose writes with clarity and authority, and her message is one of hope and humor about an experience which is often short on both."
Gwenn Cody, LCSW, LMT, Body-centered Psychotherapist

"From Ow to Wow! takes the reader through a practical step-by-step process so that they can move forward in mastering their pain and thriving. An essential read!"
Jill Fancher, PhD, Clinical Psychologist, Director of Pain Management Services, Evergreen Behavioral Health

"I thought I would be living in OW the rest of my life until I encountered Amber Rose. Now I'm shouting WOW to everyone I know who deals with chronic pain. She didn't try to fix or take away my pain, or push various healing products on me. Instead, through deep listening and gentle questioning, and following the guidelines in her book, she helped me successfully negotiate a new way of interacting with the pain. When I returned to my rheumatologist, even he said WOW!"
Kathleen McKern Verigin, Osteoarthritis Patient

Contents

Introduction

Living with chronic pain, that is pain that persists beyond an original injury, whether from arthritis, fibromyalgia, Central Nervous System Sensitization, Lupus, Multiple Sclerosis, or any of the other myriad of conditions, sucks! It sucks your energy, your attention, your memory, your motivation, and sometimes abilities. Chronic pain is an epidemic.

We also have an epidemic of addiction to opioids that has doctors, policy makers, and patients concerned. For patients who use opioids to help manage their pain, it is insult added to injury when they are treated with suspicion. Many people are being taken off medications that have helped them to function without being offered alternatives. Part of this is because many insurance companies do not cover other treatment options such as massage, acupuncture, and meditation which may seem like luxuries to a person without chronic pain but can be quite effective in treating pain. Because pain is complex, it can be difficult to find alternatives that work for individuals quickly.

According to American Chronic Pain Association, Inc. in 2013, finding information is easy, but finding relevant factual information that meets a particular individual's needs and educational level is not so easy. As a matter of fact, it can be darn right overwhelming! That is why I am writing this book. You can be your best advocate if you are empowered by self awareness, knowledge and have a map of the territory treatment options.

According to an Institute of Medicine Report in 2011, *Relieving Pain in America: A Blueprint for Transforming Prevention, Care, Education, and Research*, pain is a significant problem that costs society at least $560-$635 billion yearly in the U.S. This includes the total incremental cost of health care due to pain ranging between $261 to $300 billion and $297-$336 billion due to lost productivity (based on days of work missed, hours of work lost, and lower wages).

In other words, you are not alone. This problem affects 1.5 billion people worldwide. It impacts physical, social, emotional, economical and productive aspects of life. So what is the solution? On the societal level we need more awareness, research on treatments and causes. We also need less stigma around pain. Pain is not dishonorable. It is a symptom—it should be value neutral like blood pressure or having the flu. We need a better understanding of how pain can be detrimental to our society and not blame the people who live with it. We are not lazy, we hurt!

On a treatment level, patients need to be seen as a whole person. We need a wholistic approach to interventions that account for the biological, psychological, and societal aspects of chronic pain. We need to have more compassionate education for practitioners and patients. We need insurance coverage for effective treatment options and ways for multidisciplinary approaches to be coordinated effectively. As we move to reduce opioid use, we must have alternative treatment. It is not okay to take away relief and not give other effective solutions.

On an individual level, it is important to have self-compassion, trust yourself, utilize support, be curious, find options that work for you, and move forward in your life. Become a 'stalker' of yourself. Develop your awareness so that you can bring that knowledge into partnership with your health care providers. Know that living with the experience of chronic pain has an impact on your brain which impacts emotions and thinking. It is not just that it hurts.

One way to deal with chronic pain is to accept it. Part of what happens with chronic pain is that our systems go into overdrive to deal with the pain. Your inflammatory response is activated to fight a real or perceived injury that the pain signals which increases pain. Our stress response is activated which increases muscle guarding, reduces blood flow into the muscles and increases the release of adrenaline which overtime increases pain and fatigue. Acceptance can lower these responses which can then lower pain.

How do you accept chronic pain? Is acceptance the same as giving up? Is that not what the doctors want to do, throw up their hands? Acceptance is powerful. It is not resignation or giving up. It is embracing life as it is in any moment. It is a process.

I like the serenity prayer as a recipe for this:

"God, grant me the serenity to accept the things I cannot change; the courage to change the things I can; and the wisdom to know the difference."

In order to have this serenity or acceptance, you need to go through a process of discernment. What can you change and/or have influence over? This is where courage comes in. The courage to hope, the courage to act, the courage to follow through in the midst of pain. What needs to be accepted in this moment that you cannot change? This is where surrender comes in. To surrender takes courage. Anger, fear, sadness and frustration does not change pain, in fact they probably make things worse. Wisdom comes from the process of discernment as you adapt, change what you can and accept what you cannot. Sometimes you may find yourself knocking your head against the wall trying to change something and find yourself with a headache. Other times you might find out that you have accepted something that you could have changed. I have found skills for visualizing cooling my head that decreases the intensity and duration of my migraines. Prior to this I had done the treatment protocol that a doctor had given me and rested until it passed. Now I can work to change it. This process is how wisdom is developed.

To say to someone that they are going to have to learn to accept the pain without showing them the tools for acceptance can be damaging. To send someone to a psychologist without explaining that there are tools that they can learn to manage and cope with the pain adds to the perception of not being believed. You can feel like you were not being taken seriously or that they think it is all in your head.

Psychologists that are trained in dealing with chronic pain can be very helpful. But if you do not know that, the message you might take away is that you are being dismissed. This comes from the cultural and societal stigma that so many face when living with chronic pain. Sometimes the health care practitioner is dismissing you because they do not have any more tools to help. Health care practitioners are people too. Most of them want to help and heal but when faced with a situation that seems out of their depth some blame the patient; some give up; some keep trying; some tell the truth that they do not know what else to try at which point they either refer or let the patient go. If you are a disempowered patient, you may find yourself resigning and giving up any hope. If you are an empowered patient, you may accept that this healthcare practitioner has run out of tools in their tool box and either look for other options or accept that for now, you have all the help you are going to get.

First, I want to say, I have been there. I have been in the deep, dark place of despair. I have suffered. I want you to know that I am talking from experience—dealing with pain in my own body, living with a partner with chronic pain, and working with others with chronic pain. Second, it is possible to thrive and to find your "Wow". Thriving and living your Wow may not make your pain go away but it will make your life much better. I know this from experience! On the other hand, it may make your pain less. I have found that promises of being pain-free is a horrible trap for when they do not work; the consequence can be disappointment and hopelessness.

This book is meant to support your unique journey in recognizing wholeness that already exists which is the definition of healing that I used in my book *Path of Heart: Personal and Planetary Healing*. These Five Steps are a framework that came from my personal experience with post-motor vehicle accident chronic pain, observations of clients, knowledge of the body/mind/spirit connection from years as a Licensed Massage Therapist, and lots of research. My approach is grounded in an understanding of the complexity of the interrelatedness of life and the connections between personal and planetary healing that came from my Master of Arts in Whole Systems Design from Antioch University Seattle.

This book explores how you can find your own path to thriving and living your Wow. I do not believe in one-size-fits-all solution. My path will not be your path. I share my story as an illustration not a prescription. My journey from Ow to Wow may be similar to yours yet the particulars will most likely be different.

It can be overwhelming to figure it out on your own. Everyone has blind spots: things that we do not see about ourselves, things that we do not even know that we do not know so we do not ask questions, and things that we forget. That is why I believe a partnership with a coach or other professional is invaluable. One who understands pain, supports your developing expertise, shares resources, creates space for you to explore options, makes decisions and supports your follow through with accountability, understanding and compassion can make your journey easier and more effective. I found my own way through this. It is not impossible, but I sure wish I had had a coach like me. It would have made my journey to thriving much quicker and with less suffering.

Are you ready to thrive? Are you willing to change your "Ow" into a "WOW"? Maybe you don't believe it is possible yet, but are you ready? Ready to look at what you can change, accept what you cannot and take your life back? Wow stands for "Willingly Observing Wonder." Are you willing to observe wonder in the midst of pain? Then it is time to take a look at the 5 Steps from Ow to WOW and make your own Thriving with Pain Plan™. It is not easy but it is doable and well worth it!

Here Are the 5 Steps From Ow to Wow:

- Step One: You are the Expert on You
- Step Two: Know Your Treatment and Pain Management Options
- Step Three: Build Your Community
- Step Four: Engage Your Passions, Purpose and Life
- Step Five: Live Mindfully and Thrive

Step One: You are the Expert on You!

No one knows you better than you. Pain is a symptom which means that only you can report on it, no one else can. As an expert on you, you are empowered and are less likely to give your power over to someone else. Instead, you work in partnership with healthcare practitioners and/or care givers. You know you are not a statistic. You trust your experience and are able to communicate it. You are curious and willing to learn. You stalk yourself in order to understand your experience even more. As the expert on you, you are able to discern what works and does not work, for you.

Step Two: Know Your Treatment and Pain Management Options!

Chronic pain is complex and multi-layered and so are treatment options. Healthcare practitioners and researchers know about the underlying processes that result in chronic pain, or at least they are learning and exploring. Allopathic medicine (Western medicine) is one approach among many. It is important to understand that pain can be a symptom of something else or it can actually be the problem itself. Treatment and cures for underlying disease processes are essential but often not sufficient to relieve the pain. A multi-prong or an all-the-above approach can be effective when they synergize for maximum relief and proactive treatment.

Step Three: Build Your Community!

Community overcomes social isolation and the stigma of chronic pain. Connections that are built on mutual respect, good communication, no assumptions and mutual support are invaluable to thriving. As you build your new community, you may find it different than before. Some people who used to be part of your community will not understand or believe your experience or they may feel uncomfortable because your connections were based on doing. Some people may surprise you with their presence. Other people who also live with chronic pain can facilitate compassion and a sense of similarity that can be healing. Remember you are not your pain so it is important to have a diverse community that supports all of you!

Four: Engage with Passion, Purpose and Life!

Wow starts with a decision. The decision to live beyond the pain and a willingness to observe wonder in your life and the world around you. Locating your passion and purpose may take time, especially if engaging your passions looks different than before. A time for grieving may be needed. Connecting with something larger than yourself through your passions, creativity, purpose and meaning is the key to thriving. This is where you move beyond survival.

Step Five: Live Mindfully and Thrive!

Living your Wow is in the journey, not the destination. Mindfulness is being present and noticing in the moment non-judgmentally. Life happens and it can be messy. You might experience flares or breakthrough pain despite treatment. With the practice of mindfulness and acceptance, you can develop an approach to life that goes with the flow instead of resisting. This may interrupt escalations of the pain cycle. Resilience and persistence supports a thriving life.

By taking these Five Steps you can live your Wow! These steps are not necessarily sequential nor a one-time solution. Instead, they are essential aspects to living a thriving life. Some of them you may already have a good handle on and others may need more attention. For example, you grow and change as you live your life. As an expert on you, you have to continue observing and learning about what is true for you. You and your pain process may change over time. Observing and tracking are important skills that add to your expertise on you. Pain may change over time with treatment, lifestyle changes and other factors. Stalking, which in an intensive period of observing and tracking, may be needed to understand the changes. These skills are essential for thriving. You do not stop using awareness even when tracking is not your focus.

These Five Steps contain the essentials for living a life of Wow. For some, pain may be relieved or managed better. This is not a "live pain-free" promise. There are many out there that work for some but not everyone. This is a program that shows you a way to live fully whether you experience pain or not and in doing so, reducing some of the conditions that perpetuate chronic pain.

When you are in pain, the natural reaction is to guard and

this triggers the inflammation process and/or amplifies the pain signal to your brain. When it is chronic pain, those reactions may increase the intensity of pain. I have a friend who likes to say he finds his feet moving away from a trigger before he is consciously aware of the source. He lives with a constant headache from the effects of a brain surgery he had years ago. Noise and vibration are two major triggers for the pain. His body responds by moving away before he is consciously aware of the noise or vibration. This serves him. He is able to leave situations quickly when he needs to because he listens to his early warning system. He is a thriver. Knowing what serves you and what does not is part of being an expert on you.

Assessment of Where You are on Your Journey

Assessing where you are right now in terms of your mastery of these steps can help you to decide where you want to begin. You may find that just reading through these questions give you an overview of the model. As you move forward in exploring these Five Steps from Ow to Wow, you may find leverage points that will catapult you forward into thriving. Look through these questions and see if there is a step that intrigues you or makes you think that there might be something there for you to work with and explore.

Step One: How empowered do you feel around dealing with pain? What triggers pain flare ups in you? Do you know what helps with pain relief and management? How do you feel when you go into your healthcare appointments? Are you curious and open to new perspectives? How confident are you in explaining your experience? Tip: **Awareness** helps you to track what is happening, allows for space to respond instead of reacting from habit and supports your ability to communicate about your experience.

Step Two: What do you use to treat the pain? What have you tried that has not worked? Do you have a diagnosis for what is causing your pain? Do you understand what it means? Are you aware of the continuum of treatment from allopathic (Western medicine), nutrition, complementary, mindfulness/meditation, acupuncture, to energy medicine? Do you have a healthcare team? Do you engage passive, active and proactive interventions? Tip: **Actions** allow you to create change, enact treatment options and are needed to live your Wow.

Step Three: Who is in your community? What quality of connections do you experience? Are you willing to ask for support and/or help? Are you able to gracefully accept support when it is offered? Do you know what you need to do for yourself? What stands in your way of building your community? Do you give support to others when you can? Tip: **Connection** allows for strength to flow by eliminating isolation, loneliness and increases power. Mutual support comes in lots of forms.

Step Four: What are you passionate about? What have you lost due to the pain? Do you engage in any creative pursuits? Are you involved with anything larger than yourself? What stops you, if you are not engaged? What does your life look like when you are living your Wow? Tip: **Intention** allows you to chart a course through your barriers and obstacles by taking aim.

Step Five: How present are you in each moment? Do you spend your time and energy wishing, wanting, demanding that something was different? What is joyful in your life? How much wonder do you recognize each day? Tip: **Mindfulness** allows you to be present in the moment without judgment or the sense of needing to fix anything; it can bring you a sense of calm, peace, kindness, and compassion.

The combination of these Steps brings together skills, intentions, and abilities that can change your life from Ow to Wow. It takes practice, patience and persistence to take these Steps in the face of chronic pain. Let's face it, being aware and mindful are challenging in our society for anyone--add in chronic pain and it increases the difficulty level. It also increases the pay off.

Since no one but you can know what it is like to live with your pain, you are the best source of information on treatment and intervention effectiveness. In order to utilize your expertise, you need to develop awareness to be able to describe symptoms and be confident in your experience. If you use distraction or stoicism as your main strategy in dealing with pain, it would be impossible to report your experience because you are not present for it. Awareness includes presence, tracking and identifying patterns. With this information you can go to healthcare practitioners as a partner.

Mindfulness brings the added advantage of calm. Your parasympathetic nervous system (relaxation response) is engaged which supports pain relief. It is paradoxical, but by being present with the pain, the pain can be reduced. Different techniques work best for different people and at different times. When I have a migraine coming on, I need to use a different technique than if my Thoracic Outlet Syndrome is activated. There are a number of techniques; find those   that work best for you. It is also common for this to change over time. For example, progressive relaxation is a technique of engaging muscles (tensing them) and then releasing them, one area at a time. This worked well for me except in my neck. I learned that this technique is contraindicated for my neck muscles due to Spasmodic Torticollis. (The technique actually can trigger more spasms.) Healing comes in a spiral so that what works for a while may need to be tweaked or a whole new approach may be needed. This again is why awareness and mindfulness are so important. Often people feel like they are playing whack-a-mole. The pain and other symptoms seem to pop up when another is dealt with.

It is easy to be directionless when you are suffering or in survival mode. You wander in despair and suffering or you strive for survival. When you are ready to thrive, you can discover your compass by exploring and identifying your intentions by asking yourself the following questions. What are your priorities? What does a life of wow look like for you? What are your values and principles you want to live your life by? Digging into deep layers of your interests, creative pursuits, meaning, and purpose can uncover, discover, and focus your intentions.

Albert Einstein:
No problem can be solved at the level of the problem.

Each step is essential but how you engage with them is unique to you. Finding your leverage point(s) that can move you toward thriving can be challenging. To put effort into areas that do not bring results can be incredibly frustrating and make any effort feel futile. I wish I had had a coach that could have supported finding those points with me. The process didn't need to be so long and lonely. I found my way to these points with support of healers, friends, research and a lot of self-reflection.

This is why I am writing this book, why I coach, and why I feel so passionately about Thriving with Pain and supporting people to find their Wow again. Pain is painful enough without having to add lots of efforts that do not improve quality of life.

Community is essential to thriving and to living your wow. You can't do it alone. Isolation and loneliness are big aspects of the social price of pain. Living in a body that hurts, that limits energy and abilities is difficult enough without taking away what we all need; human contact. Pride, independence, and ignorance can stand in the way of asking for or even accepting support when it comes. Learning that it is not only okay to ask for support and to give it when you can, is essential to thriving. Sure you may be able to survive on your own, but you will not thrive. We need outside perspectives, ideas, and connection. You are not alone. There are hundreds of millions of people around the globe that live with chronic pain.

Step One: You are an Expert on You!

No one knows your experience of pain better than you.

Living a life of Wow is based in thriving. A thriver is empowered. A thriver is proactive. A thriver lives life with passion and purpose. The first step toward thriving is to develop expertise. Expertise on yourself and your experience. No one but you can know exactly what your experience of pain is, unless you are able to communicate it. To be an expert on yourself means that you are aware of your experience by noticing how pain and interventions affect you, what triggers increased pain and what makes it better. This expertise comes from being present in the moment, observing and tracking.

If you do not develop awareness, you cannot communicate your experience. Your healthcare practitioners are flying blind and missing a vital piece to the puzzle; your experience of pain. If you cannot trust your memory and your experience, you will be at the mercy of whatever preconceptions you and your health care practitioner have. You may even believe that you are going crazy when doctors tell you that you should be getting better or that they cannot find a reason for the pain.

1

Chronic pain is not a static experience. It changes day-to-day. Everyone I have ever spoken with who lives with chronic pain says they have good days and bad days. A good day may include significant pain or it might be little to no pain. Bad days might include more pain, fatigue, or fear and it affects different arenas and dimensions of your life. What affects you to have good and bad days is not always easy to discover. A delay between cause and effect can make it more difficult to make the connections. When you ask, "What is different today?" when you are in pain, may be the wrong question. The difference might be something that happened two or three days ago, or something that did not happen. Uncovering these patterns is essential for insight into what you can impact.

Pain is scary. It is meant to be. It says, "Something is wrong!" It is meant to get our attention because it may be pointing to tissue damage or a disease process. Your body deals with acute pain like a sprinter. It runs around like the robot from "Lost in Space" yelling "Danger, danger Will Robinson!" It gets all of the adrenaline and inflammatory responses going to take care of the injury. Chronic pain is not a 100-meter race, it is a marathon. Your body may still be reacting to the pain signals in the same way but instead of being helpful, it usually gets over-reactive and the pain signals increase. Imagine someone trying to run a marathon at the pace of a sprint. Not pretty! This can lead to its own problem that is not based on the tissue damage or the original disease process. It can lead to a new problem of chronic pain—a disease of the nervous system.

When the pain after my accident increased instead of resolving, I felt scared! I did not know what was happening. I just knew my body was telling me something was wrong. I was doing everything right. I rested, got adjustments, massages, did stretches and physical therapy. I did affirmations and believed at my very core that I was going to be fine. My body should have been recovering instead of getting worse. I felt betrayed by my body.

My fear was of the unknown, of being on the outside and out of control of my body. I wanted answers. I wanted to understand what was happening and I wanted it fixed! I wanted my old life/self back. I went to the experts, doctors, to get the answers. I felt disempowered because my body was betraying me and I did not understand what was happening. It hurt. I was suffering. I was in Ow! I was a victim of the pain. My fear increased my sense of impotence. I was doing everything that I knew in order to deal with the injuries including "inner work" and still the pain increased. It was relentless.

I began to question my experience. Was I really in pain or was I crazy? I thought, "It shouldn't hurt so much!" It was when I began to develop an understanding of what was happening in my body that I began the first step toward surviving and away from suffering. Until then, I felt like a wounded animal that did not understand why it was in pain. The truth is that there are many people who end up with chronic pain from injuries. I did not do anything wrong. It happened. It is one of those things that we still do not fully understand the whys.

Knowledge equals power and self-knowledge equals self-empowerment. When I began to understand the process of chronic pain and what was happening in my body, the fear lessened. It is scary to be in a body that hurts without understanding why. Pain tells us something is wrong, that is its function. People who live with chronic pain tend to have high tolerance for pain. Living in a body that chronically says something is wrong can produce anxiety, stress, fear, and/ or anger. We all deal with the pain in different ways. One danger of chronic pain is that you may ignore new pain that is a warning sign that might be pointing to tissue damage or a disease process because of your high tolerance of pain. It is like your body has called "wolf" too many times and you are tired of listening.

As an expert on you, you move beyond this fear and victimhood. Through observing and tracking, you are able to report your experience confidently and see patterns. As an expert, you understand what the pain feels like, how it affects you, what triggers it, what makes it better and worse, and you are able to communicate effectively. You understand that communication is a two-way street. You want to make sure that what you are saying is what they are hearing. When you work with other experts—health care providers and healers who have knowledge of disease processes, pain, and treatment, you are empowered to work in partnership. You bring your day-to-day experience of pain and how it effects you and the knowledge of how you respond to treatments.

At this point there are no tests to measure pain, only how pain shows up—pain behaviors, blood pressure, functional MRIs, etc. That may change in the future since research is always happening, but it will be quite awhile before the average person has access to this "proof". For now, you are the best source of information on what you experience and how it affects you. Pain is a symptom which means only you can report it. Only you can know how and what you experience when it comes to pain. Your healthcare practitioner cannot know this. Your loved ones cannot know. Even when you feel like it is obvious, they can only know what you tell them about the pain and how it affects your life. Just as you learn to trust yourself and your experience, the better you are able to communicate, the more likely they will understand.

Why is Awareness so Important?
The Key to Expertise

Awareness comes from the act of observation. In a moment of awareness, you can see what is happening with non-attachment. The non-attachment opens a space around the experience. In that space, you can learn about your experience and you can make choices instead of reacting from habit. With practice, these choices can become proactive instead of reactive or responsive. With awareness, you develop knowledge of your pain--how it impacts you and what affects it. This knowledge and what you do with it increases your expertise. The act of observing can impact what is being observed. This is a well documented phenomenon in social sciences as well as quantum physics. For all of these reasons, awareness is key to developing your expertise.

Chronic pain is not a static experience. It changes moment-to-moment. Everyone I have ever spoken with or read about who lives with chronic pain says they have good days and bad days. Good days may include pain but for some there is little to no pain. Bad days usually include more pain which affects different dimensions of life. This fluidity is something that a simple pain scale will not convey. This is why tracking your observations is so important. What causes your good and bad days is not easy to discover.

This is because pain is complex and feedback can be delayed, especially with chronic conditions. When pain increases it is natural to try and figure out why. It can be difficult to uncover when there are delays and tipping points that are not readily identifiable. Uncovering patterns of cause and effect is essential to begin to unravel the mystery of good and bad days. The more insight you have into what is happening and what you can do to impact it, the more empowered you are. This insight begins with being present in the moment, noticing without judgment, and allowing the experience to be. When pain occurs, the natural reaction is to get away from it, not to bring your attention and awareness to it. Yet with chronic pain, that is exactly what you need. With non-attachment and practice you can move toward responsiveness from reaction and ultimately to become proactive.

As I developed expertise on myself, I found that if I listened to my body, I could do things without increasing the pain and without increasing my fatigue. With practice I began to be able to do things that did not rebound on me into more pain and fatigue the next day or week(s). Attending to my experience in the moment is how I was able to do this. It was not just what I felt in the moment. I had to draw from my awareness of patterns of affect so that I could stop before a trigger was reached. One of these patterns for me was to limit my exertion so that the pain did not gain momentum and turn up the pain cycle. I learned that the cycle of pain is harder to stop once it has momentum. Another pattern I noticed was that not enough movement increased fatigue and deep achiness which also triggered a pain cycle. Before I was aware of these patterns, the pain cycle impacted my life but I did not understand it.

Pain Cycle

I overheard a gentleman at lunch one day talking about how his hip had been really hurting for about 18 months and he did not know why. He mentioned to his lunch companion that he had been at the doctor's last month. His lunch companion asked what the doctor said about his hip, he replied, "Nothing, I forgot to bring it up." It had hurt for a year and a half but when he was in the doctor's office, it was not something he was aware enough of to bring up. He was probably focused on the questions the doctor was asking.

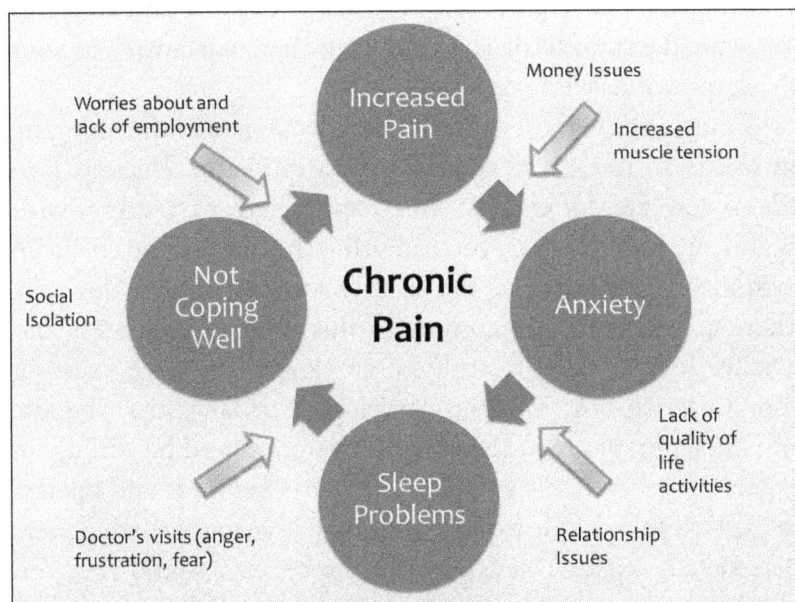

Chronic Pain Cycle

How is the doctor supposed to help if he or she does not hear about what is really happening? Maybe, in that moment, the experience of being in a doctor's appointment took his attention and awareness away from his hip, so he did not think to bring it up. Have you ever gone into a medical visit and forgot something? I know I have. Even before I was living with pain.

This man may be on his way to increased pain. He probably does not know that pain can turn into an increasing cycle of pain at the junction of nerves at the spine or that the way he compensates for the hip may be setting him up for more pain and tissue damage. Hopefully his doctor would know this but he could only use this knowledge to help if he knew his patient was experiencing pain. When you are able to see clearly what is happening in your body, you can communicate and become a partner in your health. You live with your body and your life, not your doctor. He or she only gets the snapshot(s) of your visits, tests and what you share.

Being an expert on yourself takes awareness in the moment, an ability to track, and trust in your experience. In Step Two when you are looking at treatments and partnering with healthcare practitioners, you can bring this part of the equation to find a diagnosis and the best treatment options for you. There are different dimensions to this kind of awareness and it takes several skills to truly be an expert. Presence, trusting your observations, tracking, developing a language of pain, and detachment are at the core of awareness and becoming an expert on yourself. As you develop your awareness and open it to explore your whole experience, you can recognize wholeness that already exists. You can notice the beauty around you. You can develop compassion for others and yourself. You can attend to parts of your body that do not hurt. You can be lovingly present with yourself and others in the midst of pain.

What is Pain? Discover the Territory

Pain is a sensation that is decoded by the brain and nervous system as something that signals damage or danger. It hurts. It is an individual experience that has different dimensions. It has intensity-- how much it hurts; quality--what does it feel like; annoyance--how much it bothers you; function--what are you able and not able to do because of it; and social—how it affects your relationships. These dimensions are not static nor are they exclusive. Each dimension impacts the others. For example, intensity can have an impact on how much you are annoyed by the pain and how annoyed you are can increase the intensity of the pain. Being able to pull these dimensions apart allows you to find spaces where you can have an effect and leverage points. Otherwise it is a complex experience that can be difficult to get a handle on.

Pain is a symptom. It is a signal that something is wrong. It could be a broken bone, a pinched nerve, too much of a stretch on ligaments or muscles, damaged or inflamed nerves, or extreme temperature. Chronic pain is a symptom of many different diagnoses including many forms of Arthritis, Fibromyalgia, Multiple Sclerosis, CRPS--Complex Regional Pain Syndrome – or, RSD – Reflex Sympathetic Dystrophy, TMJ – Temporal Mandibular Joint Disorder and the alphabet soup list goes on. People whose brains do not recognize pain can have injuries and not know it. For someone who lives with pain, that might seem like a great thing! But people can die from injuries because they do not have a warning signal of pain. It is important to our survival.

Pain is experienced when specific pain receptors are stimulated. Temperature, vibration, stretch, ischemia (oxygen starvation) caused by lack of blood flow, and chemicals released from damaged cells stimulating inflammation is called Nociceptive Pain. Another type of pain is Neuropathic pain which comes from within the nervous system itself. It can be caused by nerve degeneration, inflammation within the nerve, and infection. These nerves can become unstable and unpredictable. They can fire randomly and cause abnormal signals that the brain interprets as pain. This can also impact the Sympathetic Nervous System which is part of the fight/flight/freeze mechanism.

Pain affects the brain in at least three parts of the brain that have been identified:

- Somatic Sensory Cortex (Sensory Strip)
- Dorsal Lateral Prefrontal Cortex
- Anterior Singular Cortex

They work together to create the pain matrix that creates your experience and perception of pain. The first structure is the Somatic Sensory Cortex (Sensory Strip) which is a structure in the top and middle of the brain that is a map of the body. More geography is given to the most sensitive parts of the body such as face, hands, index finger, and places that experience chronic pain. This is where your brain decodes the sensory data that the nerves send. Dorsal Lateral Prefrontal Cortex is in the front of the brain and it is where pain is evaluated. In the middle of the brain is the Amygdala which scans the environment for signals of danger and threat—this is where fight/flight/freeze is triggered. Pain is perceived as danger and threat. Anterior Singular Cortex which has been linked to the emotional component of the experience of pain as agony and suffering. Pain can also have an impact on sleep, memory, and higher functions of the brain such as complex decision making. In other words, pain is complex; how we perceive it and how we evaluate it both on the sensory and emotional dimensions.

Pain grabs attention. It is like a two year-old who yells, over and over, so you can hardly hear anything else or think straight. It can take up residence in your life and can make you feel like it is all you are because it is so pervasive. But it is not yours nor is it you. It is pain--an unpleasant sensation. You are much more complex than one aspect of your experience. Even an experience as complex and all -pervasive as severe chronic pain. Awareness is not limited to your experience of pain. It includes being aware of other things in your life. Just as being around that two-year-old who is yelling does not define who you are, pain does not define you either. Pain is not all of your experience, although it can feel that way sometimes!

When developing awareness of your pain experience, it is important to observe and note intensity, location, quality, variables that affect it, and how it limits your function. These are the descriptions that help to map out the pain territory and are what your health care practitioners need to know.

First, let us look at the location of the pain. Where is the sensation? Sometimes it is very precise and localized. My elbow hurts. Sometimes it is more diffused and it is difficult to identify an exact location. I feel achy all over. Is it your leg? Where in your leg? Is it in your knee? In the front or the back? On the skin or does it feel like it is deep in the joint? Sometimes there may be different components to the pain. I often will feel pain in my shoulder joint but when I sink into the sensation, I sense tightness in my neck or between my shoulder blades. We identify the highest intensity pain first. With attention and awareness, you can identify other layers and locations of pain. As you develop this skill, you will know what to feel for and notice how to follow your awareness as you explore.

When I was a Licensed Massage Therapist, I would work on an area that was painful and be able to relieve the pain and then my clients would be able to feel another place that was painful. It felt like I was chasing the pain around their body. What I came to realize was that my client's pain awareness shifted as some of the pain resolved, other areas could be "heard " that had been hurting but were drowned out by the more intense pain. The other thing I realized was that pain in the muscular-skeletal system is interconnected. Shifting tension, increasing blood flow, and lengthening muscles impacted the connective tissue which is a continuous sheath of tissue that wraps around all the muscles and organs in the body. These shifts impact areas locally, laterally, and reflexively. I believe this same kind of interconnection is true at the emotional, psychological, and social levels as well as the biological/physical level. Even a small shift can impact the experience of agony and suffering of pain.

Next, identify and describe the quality of pain. In other words, what is the actual sensation? This is important especially when you do not know the genesis or reason for the pain. The quality gives your health care provider information as to what might be happening at the cellular and nerve level. Developing a vocabulary for the sensations is useful so that you can communicate it but it also allows you to begin to distance yourself from the experience by being an observer. As you observe, it is important to suspend judgment. The sensation just is. You as the observer identifies what the sensation feels like. Is the sensation steady or does it feel intermittent? For instance, if it is throbbing, pounding or pulsing then it would be intermittent or if it is pressing, heavy, gnawing or crushing that would be more steady. Does it shoot down your body or jump around or does it quiver? Is it sharp, stabbing or dull? Does it ache, sting, cramp or radiate? Does it feel tight, tender or binding? Is it hot, burning, tingling or numb? All of these sensations can be painful and yet each has a different quality. Does the quality change or is it fickle—sometimes stabbing, sometimes shooting and then changing to sharp?

As you explore the quality, do not worry about what it means. You are learning the language of the sensations so that you can communicate it. Once you do that, you and your health care team can identify what is causing the pain and hopefully find some treatment that can help. Metaphors can be a powerful way to describe the quality. It feels like there is a fist clenching in my low back. It is like someone has an ice pick and they are stabbing me over and over again behind my eye. It feels like I have my head in a vise and it keeps getting tighter and tighter. It feels like someone has a hot iron resting on my skin.

Next, explore the intensity of the sensation. People with chronic pain tend to experience sensations as pain much sooner than the average person—known as pain threshold. They also have a much higher tolerance of pain. In other words, people who live with chronic pain have a larger band-width of pain that they experience. Since pain is very individualized, describing intensity can be very difficult. Imagine that pain intensity can be graphed as an absolute expression. The scale goes from 0-100. Most people would not even register pain until the graph hit 30 but someone with chronic pain might register it at 10. This is the threshold. The body/mind begins to experience this sensation as pain. As the intensity goes up on the graph, the experience of pain intensity also goes up. For someone who has an "average" pain tolerance, they begin to break down physically and emotionally as it hits 70. This is intolerable, it is so intense. But the person that lives with chronic pain has adapted to higher levels of pain intensity so it is only when the scale hits 90 or 95 that the intolerable level is experienced. The intensity is the same on the graph but the experience of it is different. Still, it is the same intensity. The hammer of pain is hitting with the same force.

I burned myself the other day with steam that was coming out of my electric tea kettle. It hurt. I was aware of it and I moved to take care of it. But it was not something that I experienced as excruciating or intense. The next day or so it blistered. It was at least a second degree burn which according to WebMD is supposedly very painful. What I noticed was that my areas of chronic pain were much more noticeable and more intense than the burn pain. I don't rate my chronic pain as excruciating, it is tolerable. Excruciating and agony are aspects of the emotional component of pain. It is what the Anterior Singular Cortex evaluates, whereas, the intensity is evaluated on the Sensory Strip. Together they establish what is tolerable and what is intolerable—what brings agony. Now, days later, the burn is healing. The blister dissolved and yet the intensity of the burn pain is higher. It is now comparable to my chronic pain areas intensity. The quality is more an itch and sensitive but not a burning sensation. Yet now I am experiencing the intensity as higher. It is still below my pain tolerance, but I am more aware of it.

If someone else who did not live with chronic pain had the same intensity of pain on our imaginary graph it may have been a 70. For them the experience of the intensity would be intolerable, they may have even begun to break down. For me, the 70 was noticeable—it was painful, but it was tolerable and it did not go anywhere near my breakdown point. The itching on the other hand is more bothersome to me. It is still tolerable but it is more distracting. Maybe because itchiness is more unique in my experience and my Dorsal Lateral Prefrontal Cortex evaluates this as being more of a threat since it is an unusual sensation compared to aching. (Just conjecture on my part.)

When we come out of this "imaginary" world of a graph of absolute intensity and we look at the pain scale, it becomes apparent that each person's pain scale is unique. My 8 on a 0-10 scale (which is one that many doctors use) is not the same as an 8 for the person who was in agony with the steam burn. That is why it is important to make sure when you are communicating, you and your health care practitioner are speaking the same language. How much something hurts (intensity) can be affected by what the quality of the pain is. Let's say that I have a sharp stabbing pain that I am not used to. I have not built up a tolerance for that quality of pain. Even though it feels like the same intensity as the deep achy pain that I feel most of the time for which I have a high tolerance. If I do not understand where the pain is coming from or why it is happening, my Amygdala begins to yell, "danger, danger" because it is unfamiliar and sees it as more of a threat.

Pain is a symptom which means that it is a subjective experience. There are objective signs such as flinching, limping, grimacing that can be seen by others like your doctor or friends and family. These are known as pain behaviors which shows reflexes and reaction to pain. These behaviors do not reflect pain itself. These behaviors can actually increase pain through compensation and muscle tensing. There are physiological responses to pain such as higher blood pressure, inflammation, stress hormones released. Pain is an unpleasant sensation that no one but you can report. I have seen stoic people who have no outward pain expressions but when I talked with them about their experience, report high levels of pain. The emotional and mental aspects of pain are also very important. High levels of fear or stress can increase the experience of pain. Since this is subjective, only you can report the physical sensations, the emotional and mental impact of pain on you.

When a healthcare practitioner asks you about pain, they are looking to be able to understand the subjective experience in an objective way. To be able to evaluate the effectiveness of their treatments, they need to be able to evaluate outcomes. This can be incredibly difficult when you're looking at the complex situations such as chronic pain. Pain is a physiological, psychological and sociological experience. It affects every level of your life. It is important that you are communicating well. Intensity, quality, and how bothersome pain feels are interrelated. They are aspects of the pain experience and each has a part of the answer of the pain puzzle. What are you experiencing? How intense is it? Where is it? Are you bothered by it? Are you afraid? Are you depressed? Are you able to focus on anything else? How is it affecting your mood? Does it stop you from being able to do hobbies, your job, tasks of daily living? Is it affecting your family life and/or your social life?

Many tools that doctors use to communicate about pain lumps many of these aspects into one scale. There is a face scale which completely confused me when I began my chronic pain journey. It tied pain levels, function and emotions together. The face represents how annoying and bothersome the pain experience is and the numbers represent the intensity and how much pain interferes with function. They are connected but the tool only asks you to report one measurement—a number. As I became more of an expert on myself, I was able to separate the dimensions of my experience of pain and found how inaccurate and misleading these scales can be. I then was able to share the different aspects with my healthcare providers. I hear from most of my clients that they hate the pain scales. I think part of it is because the scales are too simplified not taking into account the complexity of what it is like to live with pain nor how it changes over time. This gives incomplete information to your healthcare practitioner.

Teasing out these different aspects and rating your pain along the spectrums of intensity, quality, function and mood gives a more accurate and complete picture of your experience. Just because I am good at not allowing pain to bother me and impact my mood, it should not change how I report the intensity and quality of pain. Some days a low intensity ache can be very bothersome. It has an effect on my mood and I can get grumpy and irritable. On another day that same level of intensity does not bother me. The intensity of the pain does not always coincide with the faces that belong to the emotions or the function in a pain scale. I can experience pain at an intensity level of 7 and be able to do most of my daily activities and be laughing. Right now the burn on my arm is at a 6 or 7 but I am able to breathe through it and still focus on writing. I can experience intense pain but not let it bother me, in other words, not suffer.

I have noticed variables that impact my pain and that I have found useful to track. Writing observations down is a great tool for recognizing patterns over time. Weather including temperature, humidity, barometric pressure changes; food including time of day, amount and kind; exercise including form, time and intensity; activities including posture, non-activity; movement; self-talk including negative statements, affirmations and repetitive thoughts; emotions including depression, joy, hopefulness, connection, despair and laughter; sleep including amount, depth, dreams and time of day; and social interactions can impact different aspects of pain. Understanding these connections has increased my expertise and allowed me to live a life with awareness, knowledge and power.

To be able to communicate, you need to understand your experience and develop a vocabulary. When you say, "It hurts!" it is not enough information on which to base a diagnosis or treatment. Remember that pain can be a symptom of disease or tissue damage and the language of pain speaks volumes as to what is wrong. A stabbing pain is different than shooting or burning pain. In the language of pain, intensity is the noun; quality the adjective; bothersome is the adverb; and function is the verb. Vocabulary is developed when you bring awareness to your present experience. It takes time to become fluent and it takes willingness. Willingness to be present and to speak your experience.

The experience of pain is complex so to begin to communicate about it you need to develop a vocabulary that addresses the different aspects, one at a time. Looking at the physiological aspect, here are some questions to answer. What is the quality of pain? Is it a consistent deep ache or consistent burning? Is it an intermittent experience of stinging? The quality of pain gives the healthcare practitioner information that is important in understanding possible pathways of the pain. Understanding the pain from this perspective can give healthcare practitioners insights into treatment options.

Pain also has psychological aspects that impact quality of life. How does pain affect your thoughts and your moods? Do you see yourself as broken or as whole? Is pain part of your experience or has it taken up the whole foreground and now it is all that you can think about and how you identify?

Pain also has a sociological aspect. One of the biggest issues that can impact quality of life is social isolation. Pain can shrink your world and in this smaller world, you can feel separated. Part of this comes from conserving energy and not having much for social obligations. Some comes from the stigma that chronic pain has. Many people lose family and friends because they are not believed. I believe that many also deal with an internalized stigma that gets in the way of reaching out and connecting.

I have experienced chronic pain. This experience has impacted my life on numerous levels. I no longer practice massage therapy. I no longer go out dancing or on hikes without considering my energy levels and plan for activities in the next day or week. I no longer take for granted that I can recover quickly or that I can sleep well. I now have a deep compassion and empathy for others who live with chronic pain and other health issues. I have developed a deeper capacity for presence with myself, friends, partner and my clients. I have developed an even stronger sense of spirituality which shows up as having a relationship with something larger than myself which is beyond my mental comprehension. I have developed a sense of mission and purpose that has grown out of my experience of life-changing chronic pain. The pain has had an effect on my life. It contracted my world for a long time and took many things away that I grieved. Now it has blessed my life with a sense of thriving and awe.

How to Develop Awareness? Witness Your Experience

Presence, trusting your observations, tracking, developing a language of pain, and detachment are at the core of awareness. My sacred witness is available to me in each breath. So is yours! When I close my eyes and take a deep breath in and bring my attention into myself, I have access to this part of me which is set aside from ordinary consciousness. It is that part that knows that I know. It is the "I am that I am" within me. We all have it. It takes practice to develop the trust to listen to it. It is the place that serenity resides. It is the source of true wisdom and not of knowledge. It sees what is and does not judge nor does it react. It is pure presence.

There are many tools to help you to develop presence. Mindfulness and meditation practices come from all cultures and traditions. If you have a religious tradition that you follow, use the tools from that tradition. I heard the Dali Lama speak once in Portland. He exuded joy and he said many wonderful things about joy, happiness and life. One thing really struck me. He said do not look outside your religious tradition to find the key. You do not need to convert to some other faith but

19

instead delve into your religious tradition, especially the mystic traditions. Each religion has answers to how to find inner-joy. If you are an atheist, or an agnostic who does not have ties to a particular faith, you can use any number of secular practices. What is most important is finding a sense of peace, non-judgment and awareness. What you are contacting is you. That part of you that is pure consciousness without the baggage of judgment, fear or past. From this place, you can notice and become aware--aware of your experience physically, emotionally, mentally and spiritually.

Cultivating your ability to dispassionately witness your experience can move you beyond the automatic responses of your body/mind. For centuries, Yogis and other practitioners have been able to develop the abilities to control blood pressure, respiration and other body processes (the territory of the Autonomic Nervous System.) Today you can use bio-feedback or training with a Functional MRI to give an outside reflection of your inner experience. This outside feedback validates your experience of your inner knowing. This can increase trust in your experience even when you are away from the machines. You do not need those tools, but for many it can accelerate the process of presence, power and trust.

Awareness and mindfulness are essential skills in developing your sacred witness; the place of knowing within you that stands above reaction, longing for things to be different and fear. Pain is something that we do not want to experience. It is by definition, unpleasant. It signals that something is wrong and our body/mind reacts accordingly. When it is acute pain that is reflective of the tissue damage such as burning or pulling a muscle or tearing of the ligament or breaking a bone, our bodies react with adrenaline, inflammation, and guarding. When the Sympathetic Nervous System is engaged, pain is lessened. These are survival mechanisms that set you up for healing and getting away from the source of danger but when the pain is chronic, those same mechanisms increase the pain and turns into a reinforcing cycle of pain. You need to go against your natural reactions in order to stop the cycle. Instead of holding your breath, breathe into the pain. Instead of allowing your Sympathetic Nervous System (fight or flight) to go awry, activate the Parasympathetic Nervous System (rest and digest.) The Parasympathetic Nervous System is also known as the "Relaxation Response."

It is difficult to feel empowered when you want to run away from your body. Pain is not a neutral experience. In order to experience pain and bypass this natural reaction, you need to develop patience, the ability to relax, and attend. It takes practice, patience and power to do this. Your sacred witness increases your personal power. The power that comes from the knowledge of what you can influence and the ability to choose your response. This is how the self-awareness and empowerment are developed.

Pain is something that we are programed to avoid. When our bodies experience pain we protect; our fight, flight, or freeze mechanism gets triggered. This is automatic. How can you change an automatic response that can have a cascading effect in your body/mind? Remember, these responses are essential for short term survival. You reflexively move your hand away from a hot oven; white blood cells flow into the area creating inflammation, and adrenaline courses through your system which are all important and useful mechanisms. Yet these same protective mechanisms can get into a feedback loop that spirals higher and higher and when the pain is chronic these same reactions can move into an ever increasing pain cycle that feeds on itself. STOP. The first step is to stop the automatic reactions so that you can understand what is happening.

Your sacred witness is a part of you that is set aside from the ordinary experience. Once you develop this ability you can access this knowing, this perspective in the middle of the day in a crowded room or wherever you are. To get to that level, you must first practice being present in a quiet, set aside place. I said earlier to go with your own traditions and now I am going to share how I have done it and how some of my clients have achieved this.

Breath. It is a powerful tool for developing presence. We breathe in and out all the time; sometimes deeply, sometimes shallowly, sometimes slowly, or loudly (snoring.) Breath is a wonderful connection between inside and outside and it is available all the time. Bringing your attention to your breath, without judging it, allows you to develop the skill of noticing. Noticing is dispassionate attention or presence.

Part of not owning the pain as "mine" is allowing a distance from it. With that distance, you can witness your experience and report on it and approach your pain management and healthcare providers from a place of strength. If something needs to be fixed, it is not "me" that needs to be fixed, it is the pain and/or the underlying cause of the pain. This distance allows you to know the truth that you are not your pain. As a matter of fact, it is not even your pain. Sensations that your brain recognizes as pain is what you are experiencing. Not taking the pain personally allows you to avoid some of the chronic pain stigma. If the pain is not yours personally, you do not need to own the stigma of the pain for yourself.

Breathing is life. As you take your breath back, you take your life back too! It gives you access to the relaxation response that interrupts the stress which increases pain, it brings oxygen to your brain and your body, it brings nutrients to your cells so they can heal. Remember to Breathe!

Awareness

Awareness is the key skill of being an expert. You must be present with your experience which means that you pay attention to all of the dimensions of it, including the pain. Then you gain perspective by stepping back into your awareness, so you can witness your experience. As you do this you develop expertise on yourself by naming your experience and getting to know the language of pain. Being aware of your experience when you are in the middle of it can give you great lessons. Here is a story of being reminded of this.

I was on my roof cleaning the gutters. This alone is cause for celebration. I felt strong enough and steady enough to be doing it. What was so amazing was the vivid lesson about my reaction to pain that I received from an unlikely ally, a yellow jacket.

I was cleaning out the gutter, minding my own business when I hear a very distinct and close BUZZ, BUZZ, BUZZ! A yellow jacket was buzzing around my head and near my face. I freaked! Thoughts ran through my mind, "I could fall if I get stung, I could lose an eye! I'll make it angry if I swipe at it." It took everything I had to just stay still and shut my eyes. My whole body was rigid with fear but I stayed still. I tried to breathe to let some of the fear go. After what seemed like an eternity the buzzing faded and stopped.

Do yellow jackets sense fear? Are they attracted by it? Or was it the bright orange latex gloves I was wearing? I have no idea but as I felt into my body I realized that I was reacting just like I do when pain buzzes by. All the possible horrible things that could happen jumped into my mind. All of my muscles went rigid with fear, my breathing was shallow—I held my breath for a while, and my attention was completely focused on the buzzing and the what-ifs.

This was a natural reaction but not very useful! I flashed on this metaphor and decided that my reaction set me up for more pain—in this case a sting. Letting go of the fearful reaction might help. I felt proud that I noticed this. I pondered my wisdom.

Just then, Buzz, Buzz, Buzz and my theory was put to the test. I took a deep breath—through my nose—I didn't want the yellow jacket in my mouth! Yes, I had that thought which made letting go of the fear more difficult. I unclenched my face and attempted not to get so tense. This was more difficult when I could hear the buzzing near my face. The buzzing went away after a while and I had successfully kept breathing.

We went through a few more rounds—my new teacher the yellow jacket and I. Each time I breathed I remembered that fear was not going to help and was finally able to not tense up. I felt proud that I had overcome.

Oh, what a great metaphor and teac—DANG! All of a sudden out of the gutter came a bee as I reached in. Scared the #@#@%& out of me. All that mindfulness and all that breathing blown in an instant. Just like my pain, when it comes at me so suddenly and out of the blue. Bam! I was able to take a deep breath and release some of the adrenaline with muttering. (Swearing has actually been shown to help with pain relief.) A visceral reminder of my not being in control. Because I was working on my mindfulness and reactivity I recovered quite quickly.

Buzz, buzz, buzz came again and again, while I worked to finish up the gutters and the more dangerous task of pruning the tree from the roof. My reactions were less and less intense. I thought to myself, "I mean worse case scenario I would get stung—I'm not allergic. I could get down the ladder and put a poultice on it as long as I do not panic up here and lose my balance."

I was warned by the buzzing sound, most of the time! I had my tools of breathing, releasing fear, relaxing my muscles through awareness, and my desire for clean gutters. These tools allowed me to clean the gutters without pain increasing. Comparing the buzz of the yellow jacket to the fear that comes with pain allowed me to learn lessons I can use with my chronic pain! I know many of my triggers but sometimes it does come out of nowhere. Using my breath, conscious relaxation, challenging my fearful thoughts and being engaged with life with goals and purpose all help me to thrive with pain. Thank you yellow jacket for the reminders!

Allowing your awareness to include your body when you are used to chronic pain can be scary. Allowing yourself to be aware of sensations that can include pain without judging or trying to fix it, can be very empowering. If you are not listening to your body, you are missing out on hearing what your body is telling you and knowing what affects it for better and worse. Avoidance is a strategy that can help sometimes yet, as with any strategy, it has limitations. Habits of guarding, moving, and reacting can increase pain and set up another turn of the cycle of pain. Fear is part of the human condition and it is natural to be afraid of pain. In order to achieve anything, we must be willing to be uncomfortable, to face the unknown. Some people are able to overcome fear by facing it and some people make fear grow by focusing on the fear and catastrophizing. The balance of awareness is facing the present without the need to fix or change something in that moment. To be aware of the fear but not let the fear block you. Awareness itself opens up the door to being able to know what your experience is.

From my Journal—Three Years into Living With Chronic Pain

I tell myself I am, I am here. I am barely awake this morning but I am aware of life. The ticking of the clocks; the creaks of the house and the pitter patter of the dogs' nails. To get up this morning is scary; so much to lose and so much to gain. When I get up, I know what kind of pain day it will be. I live with chronic pain. It is my constant companion. It is my monster under the bed; in the closet; in the gym. Or maybe I should say my fire-breathing Dragon. How do I face my Dragon every morning? I face it with my morning breath. Like many dragons, my Dragon is unpredictable, stealthy, and sneaky. What are my weapons? First, my breath – – fear takes my breath away, so I become the master of my own breath. Second, my mind attention – – to be present in each moment allows me to be flexible, resilient, and aware. These two work together-- through my breath I am able to be more present. When I face my Dragon (pain), it becomes smaller than when I try to ignore it.

I did not sleep well at all last night; I got up and went upstairs. Played solitaire games on my computer for an hour and a half. I needed the distraction but now my shoulder and neck are burning from a deep ache. I want so much to move into my life again. I see my partner with a renewed life; I'm so happy for her, and envious. I am glad that she has figured out what she wanted and went for it. I wanted her to! Yet I am envious because I want to know I can have my life back again and that I can move with ease and be successful. Right now that seems like a long-off dream.

What do Patterns Have to do With it? Key Skills of Self-Stalking

When I talk about stalking, I am referring to the discipline of self-awareness from the perspective of your sacred witness. The second part of becoming an expert on yourself is to define and articulate your vocabulary about pain and your experience. Once you have developed your awareness and trust it, you need to be able to communicate it. Many doctors use certain tools to work with patients such as scales and inventories. It is helpful to be consistent with a scale as much as possible, explain your ratings, and use metaphors so that your supporters and healthcare providers can understand. Remember that healthcare providers measure their success by outcomes. Is your pain less, do you have more function, are the side-effects of the treatment tolerable?

If you have ever had someone ask you a bunch of questions about pain, sleep, eating habits, and exercise/movement and you didn't know what to say, you are not alone. I have been there. I call it the deer caught in the headlights pose. I can remember only what I had been paying attention to. It can be difficult to remember how many migraines I had in a month. I might remember one really bad night of sleep or another night where I slept for 10 hours but to say on average how I am sleeping is beyond my memory. What did I have for lunch last Tuesday? It is easy to go unconscious about these things. I know that I have felt incredibly lost especially when I was dealing with a lot of fatigue, memory issues, and pain.

Pain is complex with many variables affecting it. In order to recognize patterns, you need to record your experience and track different variables that might affect it such as weather, food, activity, etc. Becoming an expert on yourself takes more than being aware and developing vocabulary. It takes connecting the dots of cause and effect. You can use many tools to track it including journals, pain diaries, movement, exercise, mood and pain management apps and then look back and see patterns. Recording your experience allows you to look back with clear eyes and identify patterns and maybe even see cause and effect. Using a tracking tool also supports developing and discerning your language around pain. It helps you to become more consistent with your language. Is it really burning or throbbing? Is the pain that more intense or is it the fact that I am stressed and irritable. It is also a great tool for working with your health team. They can see some of the patterns as well.

It can be difficult to remember what to do to take care of myself when pain and fatigue are high because I can get caught up in the woe-is-me. The pre-frontal cortex where decisions are made is impaired." That is why I am so grateful for my support people who can help me to remember. Mindfulness, that special kind of awareness that is in the moment and does not judge, will allow you to bring your real experience to the table. With mindfulness, you can notice what makes pain worse, what relieves it, and what makes it better. When you add self-stalking skills you add the intention of presence with the ability to track patterns and connect the dots so that you can see what effects each other and what happens and changes overtime.

First you need to explore tools that will help you to record pain (the quality, intensity, how annoying, and functional interruptions), your emotions/thoughts, what you eat, activities, environment, interventions and treatments. This gives you two invaluable things. One, it gives you and your doctor something real to look at together. (It is so frustrating for everyone when it comes appointment time you are asked, "How have you been feeling?", and you can't remember anything significant to report. I always remembered on my drive home.) Second, it gives you an objective way to see how different interventions really do or do not work.

The journal can be simple or more elaborate depending on your style. It can be old school—paper and pen, or new school—online apps. (A resource list is in the appendix or you can look at *www.thrivingwithpain.com/resources* on my website for different tools.) You can use free online software, paper journals, make your own journal, or make notations on your calendar. Many online tools and apps have reports that allow you to graph your data. It is amazing to see how moods, thoughts, food, behaviors, and weather can impact different aspects of pain.

To be a true expert you need to track things that will help you to recognize the wholeness that already exists. Laughter is great medicine. Do you know how often you laugh? What do you do for fun? Living with a chronic illness and pain can be very serious business. To heal you must use all the tools at your disposal. This includes pain relief through positivity not just anesthetics. What do you do that supports your wholeness? Do you look up and see the beauty? Do you make sure that you are surrounding yourself with things that you love? For me, nature, my partner, my dogs, and funny movies helped keep me balanced in the beginning. Now I include hiking, gardening, playing with my dogs, playing my guitar or keyboards, going out to eat, fantasy novels, and heart-warming movies and television.

I remember coming home one day and seeing three dear in our yard and a couple of rabbits on our driveway. We stopped and just took in the majesty of these creatures lit by our head lights. I could feel myself breathing deeply, reflexively. I didn't try to do deep breathing, it just happened when I observed with wonder. What are the things that make you stop and breathe deeply?

As you make tracking a habit, you can become a self-stalker. As a stalker you know what is important to pay attention to, you see patterns, notice how well interventions effect pain intensity, "bothersomeness", and quality levels; notice triggers, can tell when positive behaviors are habitual and no longer need to be tracked. Since chronic pain is so complex, it can be overwhelming to try to track everything all at once, especially in the beginning. Becoming an expert and a self stalker takes time and practice. I recommend making SMARTER goals (see the Thriving with Pain Plan™ section) around tracking. Decide on two or three specific variables that you are interested in exploring. Set aside one to three specific times a day for two to four weeks. Make sure that you are committed to whatever you set the goal for. It is better to commit to once a day if you know that three times is just unrealistic for you. If you are going to be doing it once a day, be specific; will it be in the morning or evening? Make your plan as concrete as you can. If you make the plan for the morning but you forget, do it at a later time and do it in the morning the next day.

Recording at least twice a day is helpful when you are looking for patterns that might reveal differences between time of day. Do you have more achiness in the morning or the evening? Are you waking refreshed or exhausted? How do you feel right after exercise as well as the next day? How is a particular intervention affecting you? You might have a sense that something is helping or hurting, but having it documented can really help you to communicate that more confidently to your health partners.

Self-stalking helps with awareness of delayed responses. Our bodies are amazing and complex. I remember so often in the first few years of living with chronic pain, I would feel better or worse and I did not know why. It was crazy making. What I discovered was that my body reacted to things with a delayed feedback loop. The trigger happened yesterday or two days ago, but the pain increased today and I had not connected the dots. Sometimes interventions and treatment results are also delayed. This is true with almost anything except some bodywork, pain medication, ice and heat. Other types of medication usually take a little while to build up in your system before it starts to work and many other treatment options take time to work.

Making these connections can help you to decide if something is worth the expense and risks or not. You need to give it enough time to be able to see results. Pacing, activity levels, lifestyle changes can have an impact on chronic pain and also your quality of life. It is a dynamic balance as you move from suffering to surviving to thriving. The organizing principle in your life will shift from avoiding pain, to living despite pain, to embracing life in all its dimensions. Of course we are human and so we have days that are better than others. Overall, we have an approach to life and how we respond. Are you living in an Ow state or are you living in a Wow state?

Pain can be affected by interactions of multiple variables. One of the reasons I believe that chronic pain is so complex is because it is not due to one cause but as a result of a myriad of processes that mutually affect and cause each other. These variables synergize so that the total effect is greater than the sum of the parts. In order to have an effect that increases your quality of life, you need to find the triggers that will have the biggest impact without having other parts reacting to keep the status quo.

As I look back on my chronic pain journey and look at how I live my Wow today, I know that it is not any one thing that made it happen. Instead it is the combination of many interventions, life-style changes, and treatments that changed over time. What worked for a while later became a detriment, although it was important at the time. For example, it was important for me to take pain medication on a daily basis to interrupt the pain cycle before it could get going. This allowed me to engage with activities that brought me joy and helped me to condition my muscles. Overtime, I no longer needed to be taking the pain medication on a regular basis because I had made life-style changes and attitude changes that made it no longer necessary. At this point, I have been able to pivot to the thriving cycle in order to interrupt the pain cycle and so I rarely need pain medication. It was an important intervention for me though. It gave me both the space to develop expertise and to change behaviors that allowed me to develop into a thriver. Another example was taking sleep medication. It helped me to feel the difference between exhaustion and restorative sleep. I found out what I had been missing. A few years later I found that the sleep medication became a hindrance for true restorative sleep due to the side effects. By the time I stopped using them, I was able to get restorative sleep with good sleep hygiene. A few years later, I found out that I had sleep apnea and delayed sleep disorder. With a C-Pap machine, melatonin and honoring my night owl clock, I am able to get great sleep again. Things change. Which is why being a self-stalker is so important! For a while I also found that regular bodywork helped my muscles relax enough to prevent spasms. Each of these interventions needed to give way as I continued on my journey. My body tended to not enter the pain cycle as much because my muscles were in better condition and I used intrinsic muscles to support efficiency and alignment. I was getting good restorative sleep and I was focusing on joy. I began more active ways to stretch and tend my muscles so that I did not need bodywork as regularly. (I still enjoy and find bodywork/massage very useful but I do not need it once or twice a week like I did.)

One of the lifestyle changes that really makes a difference for me is not eating sugar. I love sweets. Life without desserts just did not sound appealing! I know that diet has a profound effect on our bodies and how they work. I knew this and I knew that sugar has an inflammatory effect on my body yet I was loath to give it up! Finally, I decided to do a food cleanse and to see what, if anything, I was sensitive to. What I found was that eating sugar really increased my deep ache in my hips and shoulders that I experienced with Fibromyalgia. Not eating sugar helped my level of pain and then when I had sugar again—the pain came back. It was not something I would have really noticed if I had not been tracking my symptoms. It is easy to not notice subtle changes over a period of time. It took 6 weeks before I really noticed that my energy level was higher and my daily pain levels were down. It was helpful that I wrote down what my pain levels were and that I was paying attention. A delay in the effect can make it difficult to identify what is happening. When I introduced sugar back in, the effect was very noticeable within hours. When I introduced dairy it took about 4-5 days to notice a difference. When I combine these together, say in ice cream, which is one of my favorite foods, I feel the effects. But I love ice cream! So sometimes I make the choice to go for it, knowing that I will "pay for it later" but knowing that sometimes the joy of having it can out-weigh the consequences. I make sure now that I am not in a flare when I do it. Your sensitivities, the delay in consequences, and the impact may be different. A lot of research has been coming out about nutrition, our gut, inflammation, neurotransmitters and pain. The ecosystem in our gut has a much greater impact on our health than was understood fifty years ago.

Now that you have developed your awareness and have begun to stalk your symptoms and triggers you can move into a partnership with healthcare providers with more confidence and empowerment. Remember that knowledge is power and self-knowledge is self empowerment! Your skills of awareness will help you to navigate treatment options. Remember you are entering or re-entering into an arena that is full of stigma and disbelief. Come into this arena with trust in yourself, the ability to clearly communicate about your experience with pain, and tracked symptoms; this gives you a great advantage. The other thing that you can come in with is respect for yourself and a knowing that you are looking for practitioners who respect you and want to listen to your experience. If you find practitioners who do not do the above, then respect yourself enough to fire them. It is a partnership. On the other hand, it is important to respect their expertise. They may understand things that you do not. They may have an approach that might seem odd or contrary to what you think you ought to do. Listen, get educated, and make informed choices.

Exercise #1—Awareness

Setting the stage:

Turn off all electronics including your phone so that you will not be interrupted. Let any family members know that you need some uninterrupted time. Find a quiet, comfortable place where you will not be disturbed. You may need to put a sign on the door if people are used to barging in. Grab a journal to write in. You may want to light a candle or put a focal object that you can look at during this time if needed. Get into a position that feels supported but allows you to stay awake. For me, I find that I need the support of a back of a chair or a wall most of the time (although on good days I can sit on my meditation pillow without support.) Lying down is not the best because of the tendency to fall asleep but if that is the only comfortable position (or at least the most comfortable you can be with your pain) then begin with that. What is most important is that you are as comfortable as you can be so that you can focus and stay awake. When I began doing this after my accident, I tried different positions before I found the ones that worked best for me. If one does not work, try another.

Begin slowly so that you can build up this awareness muscle. To begin, set a timer for 5 minutes. That way you do not need to keep checking the clock to see if you can stop yet. If you have meditated before, you may want to do longer than 5 minutes. As you get used to this, you can increase the time. For this exercise, I would do no longer than 20 minutes.

Now it is time to begin. Close your eyes and allow yourself to just notice what this feels like. Start by exhaling and then take a deep breath through your nose. As you breathe in, count slowly. Pause when you finish inhaling. Then slowly breathe out through your mouth with pursed lips—count the same amount as you did as you took your breath. Pause. Repeat this two more times. As you breathe, allow your awareness to take in the sensations of breathing. Feel the air going in your nose, into your chest, and allow it to expand your belly. Notice the pause—what does it feel like to be in this place of rest? Feel the air move out of your lungs and out through your pursed lips. What is your count?

If you are comfortable with your eyes closed, keep them closed. If you feel uncomfortable and opening your eyes to look at the candle or focal object allows you to relax more, do that. Now continue to breathe in and out but allow your natural rhythm to happen. You may find yourself thinking about any number of things, that is okay. Just bring your attention back to your breath. Notice what it feels like to be so aware of your breath. You breathe all the time, now, in these moments, you are attending to your breath. In and out.

Are you breathing through your nose or your mouth or both? As you are breathing you might notice a place in your body that hurts. What does it feel like if you breathe into that place? Imagine that you can breathe into that place. On your next inhale, imagine that the air is coming into your nose and/or mouth down into your body to that place that you are noticing and as you breathe out, notice/ imagine that you are breathing out from that place. There is no wrong way to do this.

Now close your eyes again if they have been open and bring your attention back to your deep breathing--again inhale through your nose and count slowly to 5, pause, exhale through you mouth for a slow count of 5, pause and repeat three times. Allow yourself to notice your body, your thoughts, your emotions as you continue to breathe. When the timer goes off, slowly open your eyes and bring your attention to the focal point or candle. Slowly begin to look around the room.

When you are ready, pick up your journal and write about your experience. What do you feel when you are done? Relaxed? Anxious? Peaceful? What was it like to follow your breath and to breathe on purpose? What did you notice about your body? What kind of thoughts kept coming up? Were they about the present or were they about the past or what you needed to be doing instead of sitting on the floor just breathing?

Do this at least once a day for a week. If 5 minutes flew by, increase the time but do not exceed 20 minutes. You can do this exercise up to 3 times a day.

This exercise begins the process of setting aside time for awareness. It does not matter if your mind chatters the whole time. Just notice what it is chattering about. If you can bring your attention back to your breath, just begin to notice it again. Notice how deep breathing affects you. Does it feel weird to be breathing through your nose or your mouth? When you develop this ability you can see that what you are witnessing is not who you are.

Exercise #2—Breathing

Deep diaphragmatic breathing is an important skill. (If you have the use of your diaphragm, you can learn to do it. If you have rib issues, you might want to talk with your physician or physical therapist to see what you might need to modify.)

First Step: Find your diaphragm and breathe deeply. Notice your belly and your chest as you breathe in and then slowly breathe out. (If you have done this before and know that your belly expands and then your chest rises as you breathe in deeply, you can skip step two.)

Second Step: Lie down on your back if comfortable otherwise you can do this while sitting. Put your hand (or a light book) on your belly and one on your upper chest. Breathe out and then as you breathe in expand your belly and watch the book or hand rise, as you keep breathing in, your chest should also then rise—but your belly is still expanded. As you breathe out, feel them sink and at the end of the breath tighten your belly muscles. This should make you want to take another breath. Do this slowly and deeply 3-5 times until you can feel for sure the difference between a diaphragmatic breath and a normal shallow or belly clenched breath.

Third Step: Do this kind of breathing in whatever positions you find yourself in during the day such as driving, sitting, standing, lying down. As you change positions, make sure you know the difference of deep diaphragmatic and regular breathing. Use your hands on your belly and consciously push it away with your belly as you breathe in. This simple reinforcement can help to strengthen this skill.

Fourth Step: Put up reminders to do it 3–5 times a day. Put an alarm on your phone, post it on your mirror, tape it on your remote . . . wherever you will run into them.

Fifth Step: When you notice your emotions going negative, you feel a surge in your pain, or when you hear self dialogue that you want to turn around, use this technique. Do at least 2-3 breaths. Allow yourself to calm your thoughts and let the relaxation response support your sense of well-being.

Exercise #3—Body Scan

This is a tool that stress reduction clinics use and it has been shown to lower pain levels. It is the next exercise in developing awareness and focuses on the skill of noticing without judging the experience. Allowing sensations to be without judging is a way to begin to tease out the "emotional" response to pain. When you can notice without getting caught up in the fear or Sympathetic Nervous System responses, you can begin to find the pause where reaction can move into response which can grow into proactive action.

This is best done in a very comfortable position but it is meant for you to stay awake. I found that when I was having a really difficult time with insomnia, this would put me right to sleep. So I recommend that you lie down but not where you normally sleep to start to get this skill developed. I still use it occasionally to help me fall asleep.

Begin by bringing your attention to your big toe on your left foot. Notice any sensation that is there. Is it warm, cool, dry, moist? Do you have a sock on? Notice the contact between your big toe and the fabric or the air. Next, allow your attention to expand and include all of your toes on your left foot. Just notice these sensations. Are they the same or different than your big toe? As you notice all of your toes on your left foot, add in the awareness of the bottom of your foot. Your awareness is encompassing all your toes and the sole of your left foot. What does that feel like? Just notice. Now add in the top of your foot and your ankle. Notice any sensations in your whole foot. Is it cool? Warm? Tight? Relaxed? Prickly?

Now bring your attention back to only the toes on your left foot and then add your right big toe. Allow your attention to focus on these 6 toes. What do you notice? Now add in all of your toes. Do you feel the blood flow? Are they warm or cool? Now bring into your awareness to your whole right foot. Feel it resting on the surface, notice anything touching it. And as you feel ready, bring back into your awareness your left foot so now you are aware of both feet. What are the sensations you feel? Does anything change as you stay with this awareness? Now bring your attention back to your left foot and begin to allow your awareness to expand up your leg. Feel the back of your calf. Is it touching anything? What does the pressure feel like? Do you feel any tension? Include your shin so that your awareness includes your whole foot and lower leg.

Allow your awareness to go up your leg so that you are attending your left knee and your thigh. Notice the front and the back of your knee and thigh. What do you notice? What sensations do you feel? Allow your attention to go deeper into your thigh so that you are aware not just of the surface but all the way from your skin to your bone. Settle into this awareness. Bring your attention now to your right foot and include that into your awareness. What do you notice as your focus widens to include your whole left leg and your right foot? Allow your awareness to travel up your right leg to include that in your attention so that you are aware of both your legs. Is there anything different between your left and right? Is there more pressure against the surface on one side than the other? Is one a different temperature? Allow your attention and your awareness to travel up into your hip, your groin, and gluteus (buttox). Again notice sensations of temperature, pressure, tension, moisture. As you focus your awareness on your hips, what are you aware of? Now allow your awareness to move up into your torso. Bring your awareness first to the front of your body and then let it sink into your body until you have included your low back and then continue to increase the area of your awareness until your whole torso is taking up your whole awareness. Just notice any sensations. Can you feel the contact between you and the surface on which you are lying? Can you feel the sensation of fabric from your clothes, or covers, or air? Now bring your attention into your shoulders, your chest. Notice any sensations of cool or warmth, tension or heaviness, just notice. Open your awareness to include your arms, down to your elbows, down to your lower arms and to your hands. Do you feel any tingling, pressure, warmth, coolness? Now focus your awareness on just your hands, feel the palms and notice each finger and thumb. Let your focus relax and take a deep breath.

Now bring your awareness to your neck, your throat. Do you notice anything on your skin? Any sensations of warmth or coolness? Is there a difference between the front and the back? While continuing to notice your neck, bring your attention up to your jaw so that your awareness encompasses your neck, throat and jaw. Notice any tension, clenching, slackness. Drop your focus on your neck and attend to your face. Notice the sensations of your breath as you breathe in and out. Notice any areas of sensations. Expand your awareness to include your ears and your scalp until your whole head has your attention. Notice any changes that may occur in sensations as you lie there.

Now you are going to slowly allow your awareness to expand and move down to include your upper body, your arms, your torso, your hips, your legs, your feet. Allow it to expand until you are aware of your whole body. Attend to the feel of your body as it touches the surface you are lying on, the air, your clothes. Notice any feelings of sensations that you are experiencing. Now let all of those sensations melt out of your awareness as you settle your awareness into your heart. Just notice the sensation of your heart beating, bringing your attention fully here. When you feel ready, open your eyes and notice the sights around you. Take a moment to write any reactions to the experience of noticing. Do you feel any different than when you started? If yes, how do you feel differently?

Step Two: Know Your Treatment and Pain Management Options!

Step Two turns toward treatment and taking action. When I first began my journey with chronic pain, before I knew it was chronic, I reached out to alternative healthcare practitioners. This was what I was used to. I was a massage therapist and I had worked in collaboration with chiropractors, acupuncturists, and psychotherapists. I went to a chiropractor, a massage therapist, and a physical therapist. After a while I realized that I was not getting better and that the chiropractic adjustments were making things worse. I experienced rebound pain from many massage—pain that increases after a delay from interventions that did not increase pain at the time. After a while when the pain did not get better, I was referred to a neurologist. He did some memory test, neurological exam and a nerve conduction tests that was very unpleasant. He diagnosed me with post-traumatic myo-facial disease, Thoracic Outlet Syndrome, and post-concussive syndrome symptoms. I went through rounds of medications; pain killers, muscle relaxants, and anti-depressants until we found a combination of medications that gave me some relief. I continued with light massage, stretching, and physical therapy.

I was referred to the Fibromyalgia Clinic at OHSU (Oregon Health State University) where I was diagnosed with Post-traumatic Fibromyalgia and I learned more about how to manage pain, fatigue, and given additional medications. The clinic uses a multidisciplinary approach. At the first appointment I saw a nurse practitioner, an occupational therapist, a physical therapist, a rheumatologist, and participated in a support group. I had a couple of follow up appointments with the occupational and physical therapists where I learned more about what I could do to take care of myself. Each practitioner had their own expertise which I learned from. I learned about the role of sleep in my pain, physical supports that could help, adaption, pacing and things to do and not do. All of which supported my shift from suffering to surviving. For example, they told me that one way to manage fatigue was to imagine a hoop skirt that started at my neck. If I could manage to do most activities within this hoop during the day, I would have more energy. In other words, get a step ladder out instead of reach over my head to do things. This helped me tremendously with my fatigue.

Learning treatment options, self-care, and ways to manage the pain and fatigue had a huge impact on my quality of life. I was able to use my awareness and self-stalking to see what really worked for me and what did not. The clinic sent the results and recommendations back to my doctors who then treated me. They did not have anything to add and were not experts on Fibromyalgia. They just did what the clinic recommended, which was great. I was able to continue the protocols including a prescription for Tramadol.

I did not want to take the pain medication, Tramadol,

unless I needed it. I would wait until the pain had really ramped up before I would take it. Through trial and error, I discovered that if I took the pain medication first thing in the morning (the way it had been prescribed) the pain cycle was interrupted before it could get momentum. With this approach, I used less pain medication then when I took it on an as needed basis. Which basically looked like me grinning and bearing it until I could no longer cope and then I would have to take 2-3 pills a day. Shifting this also set me up to be able to have the energy and motivation I needed to do movement everyday and to find that "sweet spot" where I could move enough and gain strength without causing flare-ups.

I found when I changed my eating habits and found my "sweet spot" in terms of movement and exercise, I had much less pain and more energy (at least most of the time.) I also found things that worked for self-care including meditation, hot baths, far-infrared heat, essential oils, being in nature, playing with my dog, stretching, tai chi, walking, ice, and supplements. I used massage, different types of bodywork, and acupuncture. This is not an exhaustive list. I needed different options at different times for different pain. While ice is great for an overworked "weak spot" in my body, such as my low back or shoulder, heat is better for the deep achy pain that I feel from Fibromyalgia. Cold can trigger a Fibromyalgia flare-up including a cool breeze or air conditioning, being in a cold room, or changes in weather. Ice on the back of my neck can help to lessen a migraine but I need to have a blanket on me so that I do not get cold. Again, I was able to discover my triggers and what worked because I self-stalked. I was able to see the connections between foods and flare-ups; increased achiness after a water-aerobics exercise class that was in a cooler pool then usual; and increased pain a day or two after body-work and/or over-doing.

Part of how I figured many of these things out was to learn about my different diagnoses. Migraines and Fibromyalgia do not show up exactly the same for everyone. Research helped me to understand the underlying processes and try new things. Knowing how they tend to show up in general gave me things to look for that I may not have thought about on my own. Some people with Fibromyalgia have lots of digestive issues such as Irritable Bowel Syndrome (IBS). This has not been the case for me but it has made me look at my eating habits and how that might relate to pain levels. Migraines can have a variety of triggers such as chocolate, red wine, loud noises, florescent light, hormonal shifts and sinus headaches. Triggers can also synergize. Having one by itself might not trigger a migraine but a couple together might. For instance, if I am under stress or am at particular places in my hormonal cycle, a chocolate candy can put me over the edge. But another time, the chocolate does not trigger anything other than a smile.

If you have a diagnosis, research what could effect the severity of symptoms. Since everyone is different, it is important to notice these things in yourself. What is true for someone else may not be true for you. With this knowledge I work to avoid my triggers and do what I know will help me. I cannot tolerate cool pools but for someone with Multiple Sclerosis where heat tends to spark symptoms, a cool pool would be soothing.

When you look at the whole spectrum of options of treatment, it can be overwhelming. Where do you start? Yet I have heard over and over patients saying that their doctors told them that they could not do anything for them. This can be heard as "there is nothing that can be done." This is just not true! Integrative medicine utilizes a multidisciplinary approach and seeks to empower the patient/client by addressing the biological, psychological, and sociological components of pain and educating and encouraging options for self-care. Context, meaning, and stress can have an effect on the intensity and bothersome quality of pain. We are just beginning to understand pain as a complex phenomenon.

Pain is real. According to the Health Report HLC026E published in September 2015 by the BCC Research, entitled *The Global Market for Pain Management Drugs and Devices*, the wholesale market for global pain management pharmaceuticals and devices is projected to grow to $44.3 billion in 2020. This includes pharmaceuticals and devices. Within the pharmaceuticals segment includes: narcotic pain management, non-narcotic pain management, anti-migraine treatments, anesthetics, and other drugs (including Fibromyalgia treatments). The devices cover electrotherapy stimulators, spine stimulators, other products (including electromagnetic therapies and other treatments).

This is wholesale and does not include supplements, oils, lotions, doctors, diagnostic tests, special diets, and bodywork modalities. The fact that the market for pain management is so large attests to the reality of pain and that it is big business. As a person with chronic pain, I believe in an all-the-above approach. Chronic pain is complex and it needs to be addressed from multiple angles. I do not believe in spending your precious time, energy and money on things that do not work for you. As you move through trying different treatment options, you will need to continue to stalk yourself. Notice what works and does not work and keep a record. This is why Step One is so important. Everyone is different and therefore what works can be different. You are not a statistic in a research study. You are an individual.

Knowing this can give you a sense of empowerment. Even when someone tells you what you are supposed to be experiencing, you are able to trust yourself. When someone says they have the answer and it does not work, you know that it is not the only intervention or option. You have probably already tried some treatments. More than likely you have tried many.

Take a few minutes and look at your own experience. What have you found that has given you some relief or has helped you to manage your pain? What have you tried that made it worse? What have you tried that made no difference? Sometimes it is the failures that can help point the way to more effective treatments. Sometimes you find small things that combine to create more relief. Treatments can combine for a synergistic effect.

For example, when I first began to feel some mastery over my pain it was because I had brought together a whole package of treatments, interventions, lifestyle changes. It was a combination of many small things such as wearing shoes that had good arch and ankle supports, pacing activities so that I was not engaged in any one activity for more than 20 minutes, avoiding sugar and taking supplements including vitamin D3, B complex, calcium, and magnesium. I used medication: my pain medication, first thing in the morning, every morning; a low dose anti-depressant for pain; sleep medication, Ambien; Maxalt at the first sign of a migraine; and a muscle relaxant as needed. I engaged with active stretching everyday and began to build up my activity level including walking. We got a dog and I spent hours petting and playing with him. I spent time outside in nature around our house. I received massage 2-3 times a month. It took a couple of years to discover what worked for me in the early days. I still had intense flare ups but overtime I figured out many of the triggers and learned to avoid or plan around them.

My options expanded through exploration and education and some things that helped became less useful. After awhile I realized I was dependent on the sleep medication. I was getting sleep but it was not as restorative as it could be due to the side-effects of the medication. My approaches have changed over the years. I got off the sleep medication and now take Melatonin for a Delayed Sleep Disorder that helps with my sleep rhythms. I no longer take pain medications unless I have a big flare. I no longer take muscle relaxants. I still take a low dose anti-depressant. I play with my dogs, walk, and pay attention to my pacing. I occasionally receive massage and other types of body work. I still stretch. My particular combination of treatments is not the point here. My partner and I both live with chronic pain. What works for me often does not work for her. Our body chemistries and our reactions are very different. We all are unique with our own pain journey. The point is to illustrate an approach to treatment that is marked with curiosity, experimentation, persistence, and a Healthcare team.

Often it is a matter of trial and error to find treatments that work. Just as this is frustrating and time consuming for you, the same is true for practitioners. Many practitioners do not like to work with chronic pain because it is chronic and it does not have simple solutions. They are trained to be excellent problem solvers. Imagine that you are a great problem solver. You are successful day in and day out identifying problems and solutions. It is satisfying to have the answers and to make a difference. Then someone comes along that has no cure and is complex and subjective, it can be frustrating.

Doctors and healthcare practitioners are people too. There are great ones and not so great ones. Smart and compassionate ones and callous ones. This is why developing a good relationship with your practitioners is key. A good relationship includes trust, mutual respect and clear communication. These are essential to a true partnership.

Medical doctors may be dealing with fear that they may not be able to trust their patients and therefore the subjective information that they receive. What if someone is just seeking narcotics for an addiction and are faking the pain? In the climate that we are in today, many doctors fear this. Of course there are people who are drug seekers, of course pain is a symptom and therefore subjective and so doctors cannot know if someone is lying or telling the truth. They may decide it is easier to avoid the situation all together by not taking on patients with chronic pain, or after a few trials throw up their hands and say that there is nothing else they can do. This fear combined with the stigma of chronic pain can feel like you, the patient, is being treated like a drug-seeker/ a criminal. Remember that if you have not already established a relationship the doctor does not know you. It is not personal although it may feel very personal to you!

I have heard from my health care practitioners and have heard the same story over and over again from others that, "There is nothing else I can do. You are going to have to learn to live with it." This can feel as though nothing that can be done. You just need to resign yourself to a life of pain, tough luck. What it really means is that they have run out of tools in their toolbox, or they do not see a way to make a difference in what they see as an impossible case. Maybe you will always have some pain, there are cases of intractable chronic pain, but just because one practitioner does not have an answer does not mean that you cannot increase your quality of life and have effective pain management. Also there is a huge difference between resigning and accepting which we cover more in Step Five.

Some practitioners have many tools, some just a few. Some understand that they are part of a team that includes you and other practitioners. Some will feel that they have, or must have, the answer. When they do not, they say there is nothing else to be done. Finding the right practitioners for you can take time. For many, it can be a long and difficult process. For others, it works out well from the beginning. There are too many options for treatment and new research that is being done for you to give up because of someone else's fear or lack of tools. Chronic pain is very complex because it encompasses the biological, psychological, and sociological levels and the interactions between these levels.

What to look for in Practitioners?

Conversation setting up an appointment with a new Doctor as seen on Facebook:

"What are you wanting to see the doctor for?"
"I'm looking for a compassionate Doctor to help me manage my illness and relieve my suffering."
"That's asking for a lot!"

When you go to a Health Care Practitioner, you are seeking help. You expect that their knowledge, expertise, and tools will be able to alleviate or at least treat what is hurting. You want them to make you feel better. They view you through the lens of their training and specialty. For many, they have been trained to be objective to such an extent that they see you as a problem that needs to be solved. Instead of listening to your story, they interrupt you in their effort to solve the pain problem. Chronic pain is a time intensive and complex problem to address and many doctors do not know how or want to deal with it.

For most of us who live with pain, we have very complex situations to manage. What causes pain to increase is not always clear or simple. You may be fatigued, exhausted, overweight, stressed, anxious and/or depressed. You deal with social and functional impacts of chronic pain. Friends and family who do not believe you, or who do not know how to deal with your situation, often disappear. You may deal with varying degrees of the stigma of chronic pain. You may have functional limitations due to the pain. You may be grieving the loss of the life you had before or the dream of the life that could have been. Add in the current issues around opioid medications, the complexity of pain, and suspicion on both sides of the doctor/patient relationship and you have a recipe for barriers to a trusting partnership. In addition, it can be difficult to navigate potential support and treatments to find the one(s) that will be effective for you.

A good healthcare team can make a huge difference to your quality of life. You need to know what to look for as you choose members and coordinate them. Finding a primary care person who can help you with this can be difficult. Ultimately, you are the captain of your healthcare team. This is especially true as you search for multi-disciplinary approaches. Here in Step Two, you are moving into action from the reflective awareness stance in Step One.

Allopathic specialists usually focus on a system of the body and/or a group of diseases or a kind of intervention. For instance, you might be seeing a neurologist if the issue is with nerves or you might see a Rheumatologist if they suspect you may have or have already been diagnosed with arthritis and other diseases such as Fibromyalgia, rheumatoid arthritis, gout, or osteoarthritis. Each specialty will approach you with their lens. You and the experience of chronic pain are much more complex than any one lens. For example, you may find that you have different specialists who have different opinions on what is best. A surgeon may believe that a surgery can fix what is wrong and an osteopath thinks that steroid trigger point shots will be best for you. This can be frustrating and overwhelming. This is why having a Primary Care Provider (PCP) who coordinates and collaborates is such a gem to find. It is also rare. This provider can be a doctor, a nurse practitioner, or a physician's assistant. You are ultimately responsible for choices in treatments and coordinating your care.

As you approach practitioners understand that they want to make sure, first and foremost, that the pain is not pointing to something "serious" – usually fatal. For anyone who lives with chronic pain, we know that it IS serious. But specialists know their area and want to rule out anything that could point to something that would need a different kind of intervention. Pain is a symptom and it is important to listen to it. It may be trying to give you information about what is happening in your body. Sometimes it is just telling you that your feedback loops are messed up. It can be a long and arduous journey to discern the difference. Between wait times for appointments, doing multiple tests to rule things out, and the complexity that most chronic pain entails, it can be months or even years before a diagnosis. Then there are doctors who do not believe in certain diagnoses. After all that work to finally be told you have Fibromyalgia and then have doctors dismiss you and your pain because they do not believe it exists is beyond frustrating! So how do you decide where to turn and what to do?

Finding the right practitioner for you can take time and it may take you through a number of doctors' offices. When you look at adding practitioners to your healthcare team, here are three essential qualities and questions to help you to discern if they have them.

- Mutual respect--do they believe you about your experience? Are you willing to respect their expertise? Do you respect them enough to be prepared for your appointments?
- Listening, communication--do they listen to what you are saying? Do they respect your expertise on yourself? Do you listen to their experience?
- Effective interventions--do they have treatment modalities that work for you and/or referrals? Do you follow through with treatment plans?

No matter what discipline or treatment modality someone has to offer, can you establish mutual respect, trust, good communication, and effective treatments?

The only exception I would make with the first two criteria is if the practitioner has a treatment that you know you need and they are masters of. For instance, if I needed a surgery and the best surgeon around was willing to take my case from a referral from my doctor I trusted, then I would work with them even if the surgeon was a horrible listener and treated me like just another patient in a long assembly line of patients. I want a master with a tool I need.

A good partnership takes mutual respect, good communication, and effective actions. In this case, effective treatment options. They have treatments and expertise about the human body, disease processes, or their own modalities. Are these what you need? I have heard of people staying with doctors for years because they had the first two parts of the equation. Being heard, respected, and treated with compassion is powerful. But if they do not have effective tools or are unable to advocate for you to find other options, how are they contributing to your healthcare? I want to work in partnership with my practitioners. I also want a healthcare team that sees my healing and quality of life as the most important thing which means they are willing to work with others on the team.

As you assemble your team, it is important to develop respect for what members bring to the team. So many studies, approaches, options, theories and much research exists. No one person can hold it all. Practitioners bring their knowledge, expertise and skills to the table. Specialists know and understand deeply a piece of the complex puzzle. What is important is to find ways to treat, support self-management, and acknowledge that chronic pain is not a simple problem. If it were simple there would be a simple answer and you would not be reading this. You would be living your life to the fullest, pain-free!

Treatment and Practitioner Spectrum— Where to Turn?

In order to know where to turn, we need to look at the territory of treatment options. It is vast. A map of the territory is useful as you navigate and assemble your team. As you decide on actions, it is important to understand what options are available. We will explore the spectrum of approaches along disciplines and modalities as well as break down the level of participation that is required of you. Availability of some options differ by location. Larger metropolitan areas tend to have more options and practitioners available. This is particularly important when using passive treatment options, when you need practitioners to do something to or for you.

The following chart shows three different points on the spectrum of approaches that include Western Medicine, Alternative approaches, and Integrative approaches. This is not an exhaustive list but it does represent a variety so you can get an idea of the territory of treatment options. There are at least 112 specialties in allopathic medicine, hundreds if not thousands of different modalities and approaches in Integrative and Alternative medicine.

Western Medicine has grown out of the understanding of the body from the perspective of disease processes and interventions that rely on medication, surgery, and other treatments to treat the disease and the symptoms. According to the dictionary on the National Cancer Institute at the National Institutes of Health website, "Western medicine is a system in which medical doctors and other healthcare professionals (such as nurses, pharmacists, and therapists) treat symptoms and diseases using drugs, radiation, or surgery. Also called allopathic medicine, biomedicine, conventional medicine, mainstream medicine, and orthodox medicine." (Source: www.cancer.gov/publications/dictionaries/cancer-terms?cdrid=454743) Practitioners specialize in body systems, diseases and interventions. Western Medicine divides into specialties along body systems and intervention approaches. Allopathic physicians rely mostly on patented pharmaceutical drugs, injections, devices and surgery to treat their patients.

Alternative Medicine is defined as: "treatments that are used instead of standard treatments. Standard treatments are based on the results of scientific research and are currently accepted and widely used. Less research has been done for most types of alternative medicine. Alternative medicine may include special diets, mega-dose vitamins, herbal preparations, special teas, and magnet therapy." (Source: www.cancer.gov/publications/

dictionaries/cancer-terms?cdrid=44921) Alternative medicine is used in place of allopathic medical care. Traditional Chinese Medicine is based on meridian channels and not the western anatomical approach. Many alternative medicine options are now part of Integrative medicine since there have been studies on their effectiveness.

Integrative Medicine is defined as: "a type of medical care that combines conventional (standard) medical treatment with complementary and alternative (CAM) therapies that have been shown to be safe and to work. CAM therapies treat the mind, body, and spirit." (Source: www.cancer.gov/publications/dictionaries/cancer-terms?cdrid=689097). Integrative medicine seeks to incorporate treatment options from allopathic with alternative approaches, taking into account not only physical symptoms, but also psychological, social and spiritual aspects of health and illness. My bias is toward Integrative/Multidiscipline approach or as I call it the all-the-above and the kitchen sink approach!

Here are some landmarks to look for on your map. Just remember the map is not the territory but it can support you in reaching out for appropriate help. Each practitioner comes from their disciplines' lens so when you are seeking a diagnosis or treatments, it can be very important to go to the right specialist. These are not hard and fast categories. Chronic pain is a biological, psychological and sociological phenomenon so a strictly biological approach may not be enough. More research has been happening in the past few decades on many alternative methods which has moved them to the integrative column. I am a pragmatist when it comes to this, find what works for you!

Allopathic Medicine	Integrative Medicine	Alternative Medicine
Practitioner	**Practitioner**	**Practitioner**
Family Practitioner	Osteopath	Energy Worker
Internist	Naturopath	Healing Touch
Orthopedist	Chiropractor	Nutritionist
Pain Management	Acupuncturist	Reiki Practitioner
Functional Medicine	Massage Therapist	Hypnotherapist
General Practitioner	Nutritionist	Psychic
Rheumatologist	Biofeedback	Intuitive
Physiatrist	Counselor	
Endocrinologist	Movement Therapist	
Psychiatrist	Health Coach	
Occupational/ Physical/ Speech Therapist		
Podiatrist		
Physiotherapist		
Neurologist		
Gynecologist		
Dentist		
Orthodontist		
Dietitian		

Allopathic Medicine	Integrative Medicine	Alternative Medicine
Interventions	**Interventions**	**Interventions**
Prescription Medicines	Manual Adjustments	Healing Touch
Devices—Internal such as: Spinal Cord Stimulators & Pain Pumps	Movement Re-Education Modalities such as Alexander Technique & Feldenkrais	Vibrational Medicine
Surgery	Bodywork Modalities	Energy Work
Topical Ointments	Structural Integration	Reiki
Devices—External such as: TENS unit, Electro-stimulator	Swedish or Shiatsu Massage	Aura Clearing
Adaptive Devices such as canes etc.	Thai Massage	Breathwork
Over-the-counter medication	Hydrotherapy	Essential Oils
Cognitive Behavioral Therapy (CBT)	Acceptance Commitment Therapy (ACT)	Crystals
Endocrinologist	Homeopathy	Prayer
	Herbs	Tinctures
	AcupunctureNeedles	Hypnosis
	Music Therapy	Sound Therapy
	Supplementation	Magnet Therapy
	Meditation	Chakra Balancing
	Trigger Point Therapy	Chanting
	Yoga	
	Tai Chi	

How Engaged are You?

Another dimension to consider when exploring the territory of treatment options is the type of engagement required of you. The spectrum runs from passive, to active, to proactive. Adding this dimension is like making this a topographical map. Passive treatment is when something is done to you or for you. An active treatment or intervention requires you to actively participate. Proactive is an approach which is not in reaction to a symptom but is done to lay the groundwork for preventing a situation that increases the likelihood of symptoms; often it has a delay before results are seen. One is not better than the others. They are used for multiple reasons at different times. For example, a passive stretch is when someone else moves your body, you relax and they stretch muscle and other tissues. An active stretch is when you move your body into a stretch position. Each type of stretch is beneficial in different ways. For example, a passive stretch can increase range of motion of a joint by allowing all muscles to relax as it is stretched while an active stretch can activate the antagonist muscles (the ones that do the opposite action) to release. Stretching everyday in order to avoid muscle cramps and adhesion is proactive because you are doing it to prevent issues. This is a spectrum that can be useful to look at as you create your treatment options. Having some of each can be helpful.

Active options call upon the idea of "don't just stand there, do something!" In other words, what can you do to help to alleviate or manage the pain and other symptoms? When you engage an active option, you internalize your locus of control and are able to intervene for yourself. You are not at the mercy of someone else's schedule or whim. You are empowered and you can act! This can include things like self-massage, movement, stretching, ice, heat, meditation, visualizations or deep diaphragmatic breathing. An active option is something that requires you to engage.

Passive options call upon the idea of, "don't just do something, stand there!" We cannot do everything for ourselves. We need others who have tools (treatment) that can help us that are not do-it-yourself. (I do not want to perform surgery on myself!) When you work with a practitioner who has treatment options that are more passive, it can be scary because you are putting yourself in their hands. At the same time, it can be a relief to let go and not try to control everything. Being passive takes courage because you rely on someone else. In the case of massage and some other bodywork, you are able to let go in a way that is difficult to do on your own.

Proactive options call upon you to do something when there is no immediate trigger or relief of pain. You do not see results of proactive options right away which can make it be harder to stay motivated to follow through. When you work with a practitioner who offers proactive treatment it can be frustrating because the pain is not immediately relieved or managed. Instead, they create change slowly. This may be medications that take a while to show efficacy or it could be utilizing lifestyle changes like exercise, movement education, and diet choices which require your active participation. They may reduce pain, manage frequency of flare ups and/or breakthrough pain.

I love massage! As a former Licensed Massage Therapist, I am a fan. Many massage modalities use a combination of active and passive components. I love both for different reasons. Having a massage can trigger the relaxation response especially when you breathe deeply and take it in. Other benefits include increased circulation, muscle and fascial release, breaking up of adhesions, lymphatic drainage, and increased range-of-motion. Some massage is also active. You may be asked to assist in stretching or engaging your muscles by pushing or pulling against resistance. You can also do self-massage which is a great tool to have. Massage can also be proactive, it prevents muscle tension from building up in my neck and shoulders which helps to lessen some of my migraine triggers.

When you approach new treatments, remember the tools from Step One—awareness and stalking. By using these tools, you build trust in your experience which helps to identify effective treatments and ultimately supports you to thrive. No matter what kind of practitioners you work with—allopathic, integrative, or alternative—you are the expert on your pain experience. Each specialist or practitioner brings their knowledge, skills, and perspectives but they cannot know outcomes without you communicating your experience. A multidisciplinary team approach addresses the complexity of your chronic pain experience. A good healthcare team works together to get better results than any one member could on their own.

What Good is a Diagnosis?

Do you know the cause of your chronic pain? In other words, have you been diagnosed? Pain is a symptom of something happening to or in your body. It can be a symptom of a disease process, an injury, or some structural issue. Knowing what is wrong can give you clues as to who to go to for help. If you don't know, then it is a matter of exploration and it may take time to get a diagnosis. If you have a diagnosis, then you can concentrate on approaches that work for your disease process.

My mother had a head tremor when I was growing up.

That is what we called it. When she died, there was a pamphlet about Essential Tremor in her things. I began to have signs of this starting in my late 30's. One neurologist who was treating me for migraines diagnosed it as a familial tic. Years later, I saw another neurologist especially for the head movement and it was diagnosed as Spasmodic Torticollis. This neurologist's specialty was movement and not headaches. Even within specialties there are specialties!

So what if the diagnosis is different? What difference does it make? Each has a different explanation of what is happening, what can make it worse (contraindicated) or better, and what treatments are available. With the familial tic "diagnosis," there was no explanation other than it runs in families and no one knows why. There was no treatment offered.

With Spasmodic Torticollis there are drug treatments and Botox injections. I did a Botox injection session with the doctor who diagnosed the Spasmodic Torticollis. He gave me multiple, very painful shots in my neck. It helped with spasms, tension, and the shaking. It was amazing to feel the relief. The intensity of the shaking had gradually become more intense over the years. It was my normal. With it almost gone, I realized how much energy it took to be in perpetual motion and how tight my neck and shoulder muscles were. He also prescribed medications that were suppose to help lessen the intensity. After the injections, I took the pamphlet home with all of the risks of Botox injections. After reading the tiny print on all the risks that the pamphlet described, I decided that my quality of life was not affected enough to take the risks. I may do it again in the future--if the cost to my quality of life outweighs the risks. Maybe by then there will have been more research on the side-effects of Botox injections. My mom did Botox injections. It worked great the first time. The effects only last a few months, so when she went back for the next treatment, it did not work. I believe she tried it a couple more times with no success. (Botox injections can also be used to help reduce intensity and frequency of chronic migraines.)

One contraindication that I found out about for Torticollis is a progressive muscle relaxation technique in the effected area, neck and shoulders. This was something I had used in the past to relax. I found out that it was making my head shaking worse and increased painful muscle contractions in the neck. Because I did not have the correct diagnosis, I unwittingly made my spasms worse.

When I got my diagnosis of post-traumatic Fibromyalgia I was relieved—I wasn't crazy! It explained why I was not getting better and it validated my experience of being in pain. But then I got upset—now what? Now I have this thing; this diagnosis. It meant nothing to me until the doctor explained what was happening inside my body because of the disease process. A diagnosis gives you a place to start with understanding what is happening. Almost every diagnosis has an association or foundation that works toward researching the disease, finding a cure, supporting people with it, and advocating for more resources. Even if you have something obscure or rare, there are associations that can point you toward resources.

My body was not repairing the micro-tears that happen everyday when we use muscles. My muscles needed much longer to rest and recover and it created adhesions when they did repair. With this information I was able to change my behaviors and do more effective self-care. Massage was very important to increase circulation to aid in healing, break up adhesions, and trigger the Para-sympathetic Nervous System also known as the Relaxation Response. I focused on getting restorative sleep through sleep hygiene. I went to bed at the same time every night. I made sure the room was cool but not cold. I got rid of any outside lights. I did not have caffeine after noon. I still took naps although that is supposedly not good sleep hygiene. I was so exhausted in the afternoon that a two-hour nap gave me more energy for the evening and allowed me to go through a whole sleep cycle that included deep restorative sleep. I planned ahead to made sure that I took a couple days of rest after any bigger exertion that could create more micro tears. I stayed hydrated by drinking lots of water through out the day. The body needs ample hydration to work at its optimal capacity. According to an article posted by the Associated Press on February 24, 2016, Dr Toby Mündel and his team at Massey University in New Zealand found a link between dehydration and increased pain perception. The study was published in the *Psychophysiology Journal*.

It took me years to find my way through the maze of treatments and life-style changes that supported me to become a survivor. It took a couple more years to become a thriver. I take a wholistic approach with my clients and support them as they navigate their way toward thriving. I have been there. I understand much of the territory although not all of it. I understand the how—the skills, knowledge and attitudes that need to be developed in order to navigate treatments and self-care. I understand challenges--the pit-falls, creating a healthcare team, and the complexity of living with chronic pain. I understand how exhausting it can be to coordinate, stalk, and follow through. I understand the cycles that it takes to change. Healing is not a straight line. As a Thriving with Pain Coach, I hold a space for exploration, rejuvenation, problem solving, visioning, celebration, planning, empowerment, actions, and healing.

This is not easy. I would not be writing this book if it were.

It is an individual journey to move from suffering, to surviving, to thriving. There is no one silver bullet or answer that works for everyone. We must each find our way back to recognizing our wholeness that already exists. Even with best practices, treatments, diagnostic tests, and doctors who believe us, it is a matter of trial and error to find what works best to relieve and manage pain. Hearing about another journey may spark hope, but it is not your journey. If you do exactly what I did, it may help or it may not. What is important is the process of empowerment and discovery that comes when you pursue your self-expertise and treatment. This is what propels you from suffering to surviving.

Success

The definition of success differs. In the Western medical field, success for treating chronic pain is to balance benefits and negative side effects of treatment while getting the patient to be able to self-manage. In other words, that the pain is tolerable enough and that the patient does not come in for treatment.

This is a far cry from success in my book! It may be enough to alleviate some suffering, maybe enough to survive, but it stops short of thriving! The system is broken when the sign of success is when patients stop going to doctors. This can mean that they have lost hope that doctors have any answers. They do not see a reason to continue to ask for help. Without referrals, they may not know that there are alternatives to medication or that research is happening that is changing the landscape of understanding pain and treatment. However, it can mean that they have found some relief. With the stigma that is associated with chronic pain, it is difficult to know. That is why I believe addressing the whole person and all of the aspects that effect pain is essential. Start from where you are, look at the map of treatment and interventions in order to navigate treatments and identify resources (both internal and external). This can allow you to take your life back. As you move into the next steps, you can begin to focus on enjoying your life again and thriving.

You have a map of treatments with the topography of passive, active and proactive, a diagnosis that gives you an understanding of what you are dealing with at a biological level, tools for tracking so you can find your directions, and now it is time to find your way through the maze of options to take action!

Rate Your Treatments!

Treatment is anything that impacts the intensity, quality, bothersome, and functional aspects of living with pain and fatigue. This means the Body/Mind/Heart/Spirit are all aspects to consider. Write down all of the interventions that you have tried. This may take some time and some thought. If you have been living with pain for a while, you may have to think back. I have noticed that using combinations of interventions can increase their overall effectiveness. For instance, a massage with an essential oil blend such as *Deep Blue Blend* can help my pain by 10 (take it away) where as the massage alone would be a 7 on effectiveness and the oil alone would a 6. Often I would be out of pain completely for a day or two. The chart below shows averages for these interventions for me. At different times depending on pain and stress levels, things are more or less effective. This is not my exhaustive list but it does give you something to think about as you look at your own history.

Intervention	What did it Effect?	Effective 1-10/ Onset	Passive/Active/ Proactive	Duration
Massage from Chip (Swedish/ Deep Tissue)	Pain level of sharp shoulder pain & mood/stress	7/8	Passive	A couple days if no rebound
Aspirin (2 tablets)	Pain & inflamma-tion	2/7	Active Proactive	6 hours
Chiropractic adjustments (in the be-ginning)	Pain level & tension	8/9	Passive	1 week
Tramadol	Pain	7/8	Active	1 day
Body Scan	Stress, pain, mood	8/8	Active Proactive	1 day
Ortho-bionomy	Pain	7/5	Passive Active	1 week
Muscle relaxant	Muscle Ten-sion, pain	5/9	Active	6 hours
Zoloft (anti-depres-sant)	Mood/pain	5/1	Active	Daily I noticed how much pain relief I was getting from it when I went off.
Stretching	Muscle tension/ pain/ fatigue	7/5	Active Proactive	Built up overtime
Chiropractic Adjustments 9 months post accident	Pain	–5/6	Passive	Aggravated pain

Intervention	What did it Effect?	Effective 1-10/ Onset	Passive/Active/ Proactive	Duration
Deep Tissue Massage	Pain/tension	-4/9	Passive	Aggravated pain
Low impact water aerobics	Pain/ fatigue/ stress	7/4	Active Proactive	Ongoing built up over time, important to pace and be in warm pool
Tai Chi	Pain/ tension/ stress	6/4	Active Proactive	Built up over time, important to pace
Remove sugar from diet	Pain/fatigue	8/1	Proactive	Built up over time. The effect was so slow that I did not see a difference until it was reintroduce and in-creased my pain by 2 or 3 points.
Deep Blue Essential Oil	Pain/stress	6/9	Active	1 day
Walking	Pain/stress/ fatigue	6/5	Active Proactive	Built up over time, a couple of days.
Morning meditation	Pain/stress/ fatigue/ mood	9/7	Active Proactive	Built up over time. Trigger the relaxation response.

Intervention	What did it Effect?	Effective 1-10/ Onset	Passive/Active/ Proactive	Duration
Deep Dia-phragmatic Breathing	Stress	9/9	Active Proactive	Built up over time. Relaxation response.
Bridging	Pain	8/3	Active	Strengthen core.
Restorative Yoga	Pain/ Fatigue/ Stress/Mood	7/6	Active Proactive	Built up over time. 1 week.
Vitamin D3	Pain/Mood	4/2	Proactive	Daily
Gentle Chiropractic with Dr. White	Pain/Stress	8/5	Active Proactive	1 week or more de-pending on severity.

My partner, Rhiannon and I both live with Fibromyalgia and chronic pain from injuries but our treatment needs are different. What works for me often does not work for her and visa-a-versa. Neither one of us does well with narcotics but for different reasons. They make me nauseous, revved up, and unable to focus. I was given them when I first went to the neurologist after the accident. I tried different ones as prescribed but gave up on all of them. When I was prescribed Tramadol at the OHSU Fibromyalgia Clinic, it was a God-send. It helped to interrupt the pain cycle so that the pain did not ramp up. I did not experience the kind of side-effects that had made narcotics unworkable for me. When Rhiannon tried Tramadol, she experienced the same side-effects that make narcotics unworkable for her. Instead of helping, some of the side effects set her up for more pain.

The low dose anti-depressant also had a good effect in

subsiding the pain for me. Another thing that really helped to get on top of the pain was getting better sleep. I was always tired. If it was 6 or 12 hours in bed, it made very little difference. I was not waking refreshed. I was not getting restorative sleep. Although sleep aids are not the answer long term, they helped me to get back on track with good sleep. I added in good sleep hygiene and listened to my own internal clock. It made a huge difference in my pain and fatigue levels. If I make myself get up early, before 8 A.M., I am exhausted by early afternoon. Brain fog thick as pea soup! Waking between 9-10 A.M. tends to be my optimal time. I consciously self-stalked my sleep in order to discover these patterns. Much later I was diagnosed with Delayed Sleep Disorder which explains my optimal times for sleep. (It is a circadian rhythm disorder that means I get my deepest sleep the second half of the night and I tend to be a night owl.)

Once you have found something that brings relief, it can be terrifying if it is no longer available. This is one of the reasons why the issue of narcotics is so important. When I was using Tramadol regularly, I ran out of my prescription. I do not remember all the details of why but there was a three-day delay in getting it refilled. My doctor needed to be checked with and I was having a bad pain flare. I was in pain and distraught which made the pain worse. I wasn't addicted to the prescription, I depended on the pain relief. When it was cut off, I had a very bad pain time. My serotonin levels were affected, which made the experience even worse.

When the medication was not available, I saw just how effective it had been. It scared me to be dependent on something that someone else could take away. Many people face this issue. Except it is not just a three-day delay. When that treatment is not available, you need a plan to address the pain with different tools. Many patients are treated with suspicion and if they come across as desperate, they can be categorized as addicts, drug seekers, or even fired from a practice. For many doctors, narcotics and physical therapy are the only tools they know to offer. Most insurance in the United States does not cover other kinds of therapies for chronic pain conditions. It is unethical to take away treatment that lessens suffering without adding some other effective treatment. This is exactly where we stand today. Narcotics are being taken away often without other effective treatments being offered and/or covered. It is something that needs to be addressed at the system level. You can do your part to change the system by becoming an advocate. Check out US Pain Foundation and sign up for alerts and things that you can do. Bring your focus to your circle of influence—what you can do to take care of yourself. What do you do if you live with pain?

- Create a Health Care Team—make sure you have people who care for your health!
- Engage Active, Passive, and Pro-Active Treatment Options—move into action!
- Stalk the Results—continue developing your expertise!

Chronic pain is complex and it needs a complex approach. Just as no one thing is going to make it all better, no one approach has all of the answers. A plan that utilizes a multidisciplinary approach that acknowledges you as a whole person can be incredibly powerful. It needs to have active, passive, and pro-active approaches. You need to captain your health care team so that you are able to coordinate and utilize their expertise and optimally collaborate. Stalking the results of your treatments and identifying what you need can help you to find additional appropriate resources. When you are trying to adapt new behaviors, do it one at a time. It is easy to get overwhelmed by the complexity of the issues of pain. Do not add to the overwhelm by trying to change or track too many things at a time. Take simple but powerful actions.

What Does Teamwork Have to do With it?

A multidisciplinary approach to chronic pain brings different modalities together. A team is a group of people with important and diverse strengths, knowledge, and skills who work in collaboration with the common goal of your wellness. This can be under one roof or they can work separately and still coordinate. In this way, they can share ideas and solutions. Unfortunately, many people find that they end up doing the coordinating for themselves. This can be overwhelming and a bit like herding cats. If you can have one practitioner who acts as the coordinator, such as your family doctor or Primary Care Provider (PCP), they can encourage collaboration and aid in communication.

No matter how you organize it, you are the captain of the team. You pick the team members. You do the heavy lifting of the active treatments. When you are using your resources to focus on your healing, it can be invaluable to have team members who take up other roles. As the team captain you delegate roles to others. This is when having a great PCP, a medical advocate, or a family member who can step up is a blessing. That person can help to coordinate appointments, communication of treatments and labs, and encourage collaboration.

You bring your awareness and stalking skills to inform the team as to the effectiveness of interventions. Openness and honesty about your experience, confident self-expertise, and curiosity about different interventions set the stage for good communication which can have a huge impact on creating an effective team. You need to be able to communicate your experience in a way that your team can hear. You may be angry, frustrated or depressed but it is important to communicate respectfully. It is not your team's fault that you are in pain. Nor is it yours! Use good communication with team members. This includes listening, checking assumptions, clarity of messages (verbal and nonverbal), and respect.

Your team can include more than medical doctors. It can include massage therapists, physical therapists, counselors, acupuncturists, yoga instructors, a health coach, other practitioners, and others who support your wellness. You are an important part of the team and your family and friends can be too. (My partner goes to most of my appointments as part of my team. I do the same for her.) Some clinics actually work in a team model. Different modalities gather and coordinate care in-house. This may not be available in your area.

Some practitioners are open to a team model but may not have the time or skills to collaborate with other practitioners if they are not in such a practice. You may come up against professional rivalries, general misunderstanding or mistrust about other kinds of providers. For instance, some alternative care providers have a general mistrust of the "medical establishment" and some medical doctors can have biases against other types of providers such as chiropractors or naturopaths.

During the first year after my accident, my chiropractor played a huge role in collaborating with other practitioners by referring me and listening to what came back. After a while, I realized that the chiropractic adjustments were making things worse instead of better. He stayed an important team member because I appreciated the way he communicated respectfully, encouraged collaboration, and brought a blend of expertise and curiosity. My team has grown and changed over the past 14 years.

The roster started with myself, my partner, my chiropractor and a massage therapist. When things did not improve in the way we were expecting, a neurologist was added. Next came a physical therapist and a couple of other massage therapists. At about the ninth month, I added an attorney to help with the legal pieces of the accident who suggested a referral up to the OHSU Fibromyalgia Clinic. This added important information but the practitioners did not "join" the team. I added my primary care provider who carried out the treatment plan from the Fibromyalgia Clinic, a couple more massage therapists, and an acupuncturist. At one point my fatigue began to become almost more bothersome than the pain. I added a naturopath who supported me with my endocrine system. This helped tremendously. It was not a quick fix, it took time to get sustained results.

Over the years I have had a few PCPs—mostly due to my providers moving on from my area or my changing insurance plans. I have been fortunate in that they have all been willing to listen, respect, coordinate and collaborate. Most of them did not have much to add to the treatment of chronic pain or fatigue other than refer me to others. I have worked with integrative, alternative care and specialists who support my healing including counselors, energy healers, nutritionists, and a variety of body workers.

Exercise #4—Developing your Roster

As you move forward with building a winning healing team it is good to stop, take roll call, identify the strengths and weaknesses in your team, and plan your next steps for team development.

1. With your diagnosis are there specialists that you want on your team?
2. Who is on your team? (List providers and supporters who help with treatment and coordination.)
3. As the captain of your team, how do you encourage collaboration and coordination?
4. How can you communicate more effectively?
5. Do you have a variety of interventions that you use?
6. Do they include active and proactive options?
7. Do you have a breakthrough pain plan? (See Part Six.)
8. What resources can you find that can give you accurate information on your diagnosis?
9. What kinds of therapy do you want to try?
10. What kinds of life-style changes do you think will support your thriving?
11. How comfortable are you with your family doctor or PCP when it comes to discussing your chronic pain?
12. Who can you ask for recommendations?
13. Who can you turn to for treatment and what options are your most curious about?

Exercise #5—Rate Your Treatment History

Use the chart in the appendix or download one from www.
thrivingwithpain.com/resources. Here are some categories that
might help spark your memory.

Lifestyle Changes	Nutrition	Supplements	Medication
Activity levels	Bodywork/ Massage	Meditation	Stress Man-agement
Counseling/ Coaching	Physical Therapy	Devices	Topical Applications

Once you have identified what has already worked, you can
develop a comprehensive self-care plan that includes multiple
modalities.

- What are your top needs to be addressed (i.e. stress, mood, muscle tension, flexibility, pain intensity, bothersome level of pain, coping-skills.)
- Write down the treatments that have worked.
- Add in any treatments that you want to add.
- How are they addressing your needs?
- Identify any active and proactive approaches.
- Note what helps quickly.
- Note preventative approaches.
- Write down your plan for any breakthrough pain.

Exercise #6—Create a Pain Relief Kit

Put together a plan for your pain relief so that when the flares or break through pain comes and you cannot remember what to do, you have a place to go with all of your tools. Make a list and then put the tools all together in one place, or directions to where things are.

You may have different pains that need different kits. For instance, I have different needs for Fibromyalgia flares, migraines, Thoracic Outlet Syndrome or Torticollis. Ice makes the Fibro worse but helps migraines and Thoracic Outlet Syndrome. Your kit should have all your tools so that when you are in pain, you do not have to remember what to do! Include health care providers and contact information that you may want to make appointments with. Think of this as your first aid kit for pain!

Step Three: Build Your Community!

It is the small things that can make a big difference.

The Big No

I was exhausted and in pain. My whole body throbbed with a deep ache, my low back was in spasm, my right shoulder felt like a knife was sticking in it and my neck was exhausted from holding up my head. I felt like a deflated balloon with no air left. The thought of sitting in a restaurant and going to a movie was just too much. Another event I would need to cancel. It felt like a punch in the stomach. I told my partner I was just not up for going out but to go ahead. Just because I could not go, did not mean she could not go. I felt awful. I had been doing so well and the Big NO felt like my world was crumbling.

Rhiannon called our friends to let them know that I had to beg out, once again. I knew I was taking care of myself. I needed to rest and support my body. That did not take away the ache in the pit of my stomach that signaled disappointment, defeat and loneliness. I had looked forward to seeing our friends and the movie. But I had to balance my energy and my commitments. I was working full time and that was about all I seemed to be able to do. I was bummed to say the least!

I was in a stew of self-pity when she came back from talking with them. I tried to put on a brave face so that I could reassure her that it was fine to go out without me. I really wanted her to stay home so I did not have to feel alone but what she said changed my life. John and Stephanie were coming over and bringing pizza and a Netflix DVD. I could feel the tears leak out of my eyes. Then I felt bad, even guilty that everyone was going to miss the dinner out and the movie we had planned to see. (Now I cannot remember what movie it was.)

"Oh, you guys do not have to do that! No, no, go ahead. I do not want to be a wet blanket."

"We know that, but they said they want to see you." Rhiannon replied.

The ache in my stomach dissipated and I burst into tears of relief and joy. That evening, I sat in my lounge chair and held court, at least that was how it felt. I ate pizza, visited, laughed and watched a DVD. It was the best gift I ever received. For these friends, it was a no-brainer. They wanted to spend time with their friends, Rhiannon and myself. So when they saw a way to do it, they suggested it. I was going to eat dinner and watch television on my own if they had gone without me. So I got to take care of myself and be with supportive friends. After that, I realized that I could ask for what I needed and not feel guilty. I could trust that if it did not work for someone, they could tell me.

This was a turning point for me in my journey from a sufferer, to a survivor, to a thriver. I had made plans which is a mark of a survivor. I was not letting the pain win or shrink my world. When I canceled and then accepted their suggestion,

I moved into thriving territory. I said yes through my no and was able to gracefully, through my tears, accept the connection in another form; in instead of out, be instead of do. Later on in my journey, I took the next step which I do most of the time now. I make plans and let my friends know that I will take care of myself and that might mean I need to change things. Now instead of just cancelling, I make an alternative suggestion that I can say yes to. (Sometimes, rarely now, I reschedule.)

What I realized the night that our friends brought pizza and a movie was that it was the connection that meant the most. What we did was secondary. My community is important. They are the people I am connected to including my partner, family, friends, co-workers, neighbors, acquaintances, support group members, the health care practitioners that work with me, my dogs, my spiritual beliefs and nature. It reminds me a bit of being a teenager, just hanging out.

"What did you do?" my mom would ask.

"Nothing," I would answer.

"Well, did you have fun?"

"Yeah!"

The Social Cost of Pain

One of the most difficult issues with chronic pain is isolation. Our world can become smaller as pain and fatigue take over. We focus on what it takes to survive. The pain begins to take over and take center stage. We organize our life around it. We can lose what makes life worth living; connections. This is why the third step is community and the skill is connection.

Social isolation is a huge problem for many who live with chronic pain. As we manage our symptoms, our energy, or not manage them, it is easy to not make the effort it takes to stay connected to others. Informal connections are how many of us find each other, through workplaces, shared spaces, hobbies, etc. When our lives become smaller and smaller and when our abilities change, those same forums can go away. It takes energy to find other ways to connect. Energy that is just not available when you are suffering or trying to survive.

When you are not able to do things because of the pain, this can shift your connections with community. You may no longer be able to engage with many of the pursuits that your community is organized around and so the informal opportunities shrink. Social connections established through work and social circles are eroded due to lack of energy and/or employment loss. It is difficult to go out right after work with the gang to a happy hour or you might not be able to keep a job. After my accident, I was no longer able to do my work, massage therapy.

You may also need support in ways that you did not before. Support comes in many shapes and sizes. The kind of support my friends gave me by coming over with pizza and a movie was incredible. It may not sound like much but that small gesture of wanting connection with me was priceless. It was physical and emotional support. The chair that I sat in was a physical support that Vocational Rehabilitation got for me so that I could work at home but it also symbolized emotional and mental support because it told me that someone believed I could do it. I could work. Not the work I did before but new work, coaching instead of massage and teaching. I had given up on myself and my abilities. This chair symbolized that others believed that I could work. That supported me mentally and emotionally as much as the chair supported my body.

Support can make the difference between suffering and surviving. It can also be what catapults you into thriving. I tend toward tunnel vision when I am feeling down. If people are not in my daily life, I forget that they are still connected to me when I am feeling alone. When I stop and really think about who I am connected with, who I would help if needed and who I could imagine would be there for me, I have a lot more than the people in my day-to-day life. This is why finding and accepting support is an important step. It takes work internally and externally to connect but the rewards are amazing. Internally you need to allow yourself to understand what you need, ask for it and be willing to accept it. Externally you need to find resources, be vulnerable enough to ask, have clear communication, gracefully accept it, know that the answer may be no and recognize when you can support others. The reward is a life lived in connection and not isolation. It is a life lived to the fullest instead of a life eked out.

If you have been living in isolation or as a hermit, it can be difficult to remember who may still be out there. If you have been living the stoic life of "I can do it myself", it can be difficult to let anyone know what is really going on. If you have felt needy but not connecting, it can be difficult to believe anyone cares. Support is a manifestation of connections. My friends who brought the pizza wanted to connect. In doing that, they supported me. I, in my way, supported them by being open. I did not put up roadblocks. We connected that night. I let them know how much their actions touched me. Isolation robs you of connections that can make your life full. Connections can move you beyond suffering to surviving and connections can support thriving because they nourish your flourishing.

It can feel like no one gets it. It can be difficult to ask for help or to know who to ask. Many of us are proud and we do not like to look or feel weak. Many of us have always been the supporters and caretakers and it can be difficult to see ourselves in the role of needing. Some of us ask for support only to find that the support is not there. Many of us do not know what we need in terms of support. Friends and family are not sure what to do. We may expect people to just know how we are feeling. Sometimes others go into denial which makes it even more difficult to connect because they are denying our experience of pain. Healing is recognizing wholeness that already exists. How this relates to support is recognizing the connections that you already have and the things that make your life possible. Often when we are in pain it can be easy to miss what is already in front of us. Periodically in my life, even before chronic pain, I would get morose about how nobody liked me. I deeply felt the words to an old children's song, "Nobody Likes Me, Everybody Hates Me", also known as "I Guess I'll Go Eat Some Worms." I felt separate and alone. That was never the truth. I have always had a community of friends and family who love and support me. People who feel connected to me but there have been times that I have not been able to see it. You probably have people in your life who want to be connected, who would like to support you, but may not know how, or you may not recognize the connection. My friends who came over that night had been in my life for a couple of years but I did not realize the depth of connection that was there already. Their action of support which they did not see as anything big, opened my eyes. It also gave me the courage to ask for what I need. Getting together and spending time together was what everyone wanted. It is easy to forget that and put the emphasis on the "what" of doing. It was less scary to focus on the "doing" rather than the "being", because it was less about me. Chronic pain and fatigue can make doing less possible and therefore "being" comes to the forefront, if you let it. If you do not, you lose more than what you cannot do anymore.

Pain is scary. It is scary for people who live with it and it is scary to witness. It is especially scary to witness it in someone you care about. People deal with fear in different ways. Sometimes it shows up as denial, "If I do not acknowledge it, then I do not have to deal with it." Sometimes is shows up as anger, "If I am angry, then I do not have to deal with how out-of-control I feel." Sometimes people react by trying to fix whatever they are scared of, in this case, pain or the person in pain. They may try to give advice as to what you should do for the pain or do things for you that you can and want to do for yourself. These reactions can get in the way of connecting and giving and receiving appropriate support. This can be true for you and the people in your life. A big difference is that you are not able to leave in order to escape the source of the fear—the pain. Instead, you have to deal with it. How you deal with it can have a big impact on the connections and support in your life. This is why becoming an expert on yourself and finding effective treatments are Step One and Two.

You have needs, everyone does. According to Maslow's hierarchy of needs there is a pyramid that starts with the basic physiological needs of survival—food, shelter, air, water. The next level is safety such as personal safety, financial security, health. Then come the needs of love and belonging. Then the need of esteem in the form of respect, from self and others. Then the need for self-actualization which is realizing one's potential. Later in life Maslow added the need for self-transcendence which occurs when you give yourself to some higher purpose or goal larger than yourself. Thriving occurs when you are able to meet your basic needs while engaging with something larger than you.

In order to thrive you need to nurture your connections and accept support while giving yourself to some higher goal or purpose. It is a paradox! In order to give you must be willing to receive. In order to receive you must be willing to give. Support is a mutual exchange of energy. Yet it is not a transactional log book tally. There will be times when you need to receive support and it may seem like you have nothing to give. Just because you feel that someone is giving and you have nothing to give in return does not mean that they are not receiving. The truth is, when someone gives and it is gracefully received, they receive the gift of self-transcendence, the highest level of need. One way you can make sure that there is a mutual exchange is when you feel you have nothing to give is to not get in the way of the offered support or connection. You can give by gracefully accepting the support that is given, even if it is not exactly what you wanted, as long as it does not cross your boundaries.

We in the west live in a society that already has difficulty with connecting. People spend more time on their devices and less on being present with each other. Just look around and you will find people who are together, but not connecting. Instead they are talking or texting people on their phones. Add to this how busy people are in general and it becomes more difficult to just connect. If you lose your job due to your health situation, you lose a source of connection and a source of some of your safety needs. If you and your friends had been active and now you can no longer can do activities that you used to, you have lost an important avenue of connection. If your family or friends do not believe that you are in pain, this can impact your connection. Unfortunately, these are not unusual circumstances. Most people who had once been healthy have to adjust to a new normal and this can change who and how others are in your life. It takes work to stay connected and ask for support. Sometimes you can be surprised by the support, understanding and the connections from people who stay with you. New people show up in your life who bring new connections. On the other hand, it can be shocking to see who walks away.

How Many Bars?

The support you have may not look the way you want it to be--yet. It is like the bars on your cell phone. How connected do you feel? One bar, two bars, three bars, all the bars? One way to look at it is to become more aware of connections and taking positive steps to nurture them. Sometimes you have to go outside for a good connection or go to one side of the house. Until that night with my friends, I was muscling through. I wanted to be connected with friends and so I would do things that were not supportive of my health and then have rebound pain and fatigue. Eventually I began to take care of myself by cancelling when I felt I was not up for it. But then I felt isolated and depressed. I would get in the spiral of thinking that I was not able to be relied on which was not how I had ever seen myself before. I was surviving. I went when I could but I made fewer plans. I did not want to be the flake that always cancelled at the last minute. Instead, I became the person that could not commit.

When my friends gave me an option for a back up plan, the light went on. I did not need to live in the either/or, I could live in the both/and/plus. As I mentioned before, I began to make plans with the understanding that I may need to cancel at the last minute and we could come up with backup plans if appropriate. No more yes-or-no. It was like the roaming began to work on my cell phone. What became clear was that the connection was the most important thing. The quality of my connections became the focus and not the "what" of doing. It was scary to get to this place--to ask for what I needed without demanding or pleading. My connections became deeper. They were based on who I am and not on what I did. I was able to do more because I was willing to modify my doing and my friends were willing to come along. The increase in the quality of my life made the risk of being seen and vulnerable worth it. This was the plus!

One of the amazing results was that the more plans I made, the more I was able to! I found ways to make things more doable. Sitting on the aisle in the movie so I could stand and stretch if I needed to; bringing a jacket I could roll up and use as a lumbar support in a booth in a restaurant; asking friends to walk at my pace so I did not hurt myself. These were some strategies that made outings more enjoyable and doable. The more I connected, the more connected I felt. It was like more cell towers were put up and I had all my bars. I got energy from being with friends even when I was fatigued when I got home. The next day I would feel enlivened. Looking forward to plans also gave me energy and helped me to pace other activities.

Sources of Support

Support can come in lots of forms. It can be physical, emotional, intellectual, spiritual or all of the above. It allows you to function at your highest level, feel connected and to thrive. I facilitate a support group in Portland, Oregon once a month for Fibromyalgia, chronic pain/fatigue. We have new people almost every time: people who come for months and even years, and people who find community and then move on. We share our experiences-both our challenges and what has helped; we laugh, we cry, but most importantly we connect. We have an informal lunch that happens once a month for people to get together outside of a support group environment to have another opportunity to connect. I focus our group on the positive as much as possible without denying how difficult it can be. We also have members that are not employed, have been turned down for SSDI and who need the basics of survival. We have members who work or who are retired that want a sense of community. Members are so grateful for the companionship, understanding and resources that everyone brings. The thing that new members marvel at is the laughter. I truly believe that laughter is the best medicine for the body and soul.

Support from others who live with pain is invaluable. People sense that they do not need to explain how it feels to live with pain and fatigue—it is just a given. When you are with others who live with pain, you can have short-hand conversations. It is understood that it can take three hours in the morning just to get moving, or that flare ups can come out of the blue, and plans may need to change at the last minute. It is understood that getting to a water aerobics class a half hour late can be cause for celebration. Things that "other" people might not get, this community understands. It is okay if we laugh about these things. We are on the inside of the joke, if our families laughed, we might be offended. I overheard a couple of people in my Fibromyalgia support group laughing about how long it can take for two people with chronic pain to get together for a date since they both have to be okay on the same day! Given that hundreds of million of people live with moderate to severe chronic pain, I am sure you know people who live with pain. You may just not know it.

Physical supports can be as simple as adapting how you do things or how others do things for you. When you are able to figure out what is supportive, then you can begin to make those changes. Daily activities like grocery shopping can become mountains. Strategies to make it easier and more doable exist. Are you willing to try them? Most stores now have customer service employees who can go around with you and put things into your cart. The electric scooters can lessen the amount of energy you need to put out. I used them for a while when my fatigue and pain were really flaring up. I could walk but walking on concrete increased the pain and it was exhausting. I know I felt silly and even embarrassed but it made a difference to my ability to do other things that day. So I used it and ignored the glances as I stood up to reach for groceries to put in my cart. Even how the bags are packed is important. If you cannot lift more than 10 pounds, the bags need to be packed lightly. If you need to rest before you can put the groceries away, you need a way to keep the perishables cold or packed separately to be put away first. What happens in the store is only half the battle. The other half is getting home and getting the groceries in and put away. My partner will often leave some of the heavier items in the car to be retrieved later. You can put the perishables away or you can put an ice pack into a thermal bag. It is okay to leave the bags out and rest before you put the groceries away!

Physical support and pacing are one of the most difficult pieces of the thriving puzzle. Especially for people with Fibromyalgia, fatigue and autoimmune issues. When I have a good day I want to do more. I can over-do it if I am not conscious about my choices and I can pay for it later. On bad days, I need to be gentler with myself yet I need to do some so that I do not slip into de-conditioning. It can be difficult to find that razor's edge of pacing because it changes. That is part of why emotional and mental support is so helpful.

When I first went back to work fulltime at InsideTrack Inc. as a Success Coach, I had two people from Vocational Rehabilitation come in and support my transition. The first was a job coach who gave me tips on memory aids, explaining my communication needs and pretty much letting me know that I could do it. This moral support was important because I was not so sure at the time that I could do it. The second was an ergonomic specialist that came in and gave me recommendations about the equipment I needed and how to use it. I already had the prescription from OHSU that I needed a special chair. It had to have adjustable arms, a head rest and lots of adjustments for the seat. It became known as the "Captain's chair" like from Star Trek. It stood out among the rest of the regular chairs in cube land. I needed to change positions regularly and I was able to do that with an adjustable keyboard tray that allowed me to stand and to sit. I needed a foot rest that moved and the ability to self-regulate my energy. I worked from home midweek and coached from my recliner, which helped with fatigue. The physical supports, the recommendations from my coaches, along with the support and flexibility of my manager to let me work from home made it possible for me to work full time.

My Captain's chair stood out at the office. I was a little uncomfortable since I was new. (I had a lot of envious looks. I mean, who would not want such a comfy chair?) It felt like a miracle I was able to work at all and having a special chair that stood out was a small price. The notoriety gave me a choice, an opportunity, to educate people about chronic pain. I became the ergonomics expert and did a few workshops for the company. Many people did not have chronic pain but office work can lead to issues, so the information was preventative and proactive. I also found many people who were dealing with chronic pain who had not "come out" at work about it. I was able to help them to do their jobs with less pain. Lights above desks began to go out around the office, keyboard trays were ordered and makeshift footrests were seen under desks.

These supports made it possible for me to work and it helped others as well. The understanding of my manager and the support of my team was amazing. I was blessed to find a flexible work environment that did not seem to have the stigma associated with chronic pain. As with life, it was not a straight line. It took time for me to figure out what worked for me. I changed teams a number of times which included needing to negotiate about working from home. I did need to take medical leave during my tenure due to fatigue. It got so bad that I could not function. I was exhausted and not able to do my job. I needed naps during the day. Not short cat naps, but two hour naps just to get through the day. I could not keep my eyes open or concentrate.

I found out that sleep apnea was the culprit. I had to wait for the diagnosis and the CPAP machine before I could go back to work. I think it was 8 weeks. Taking that medical leave allowed me to keep my job. Otherwise, I would have probably been fired because I was not performing my work. Although I did not have income during this time, I felt blessed that I could figure it out and get back to work. About a year and half later, I decided that it was time for me to leave. I had figured out the rhythm that worked for me and there were no positions that would allow my schedule. I also wanted to pursue coaching in my Thriving with Pain practice.

All of this support happened because I asked for it in a proactive way and found available support. When I was denied Social Security Disability I pursued support from Vocational Rehabilitation Services. I figured out by asking experts and being self-aware about what I needed. I asked about triggers for Fibromyalgia, memory issues from post-concussive syndrome, low back and neck pain, migraines and Thoracic Outlet Syndrome (TOS) and got advice on ways to manage well.

I used the advice and then used my awareness and presence (from Step One) to adjust as needed. Persistence is a hallmark of thriving.

I used my workstation in the way I was told would be best which included varying the way I used it; I got up and down while talking to keep myself moving and my joints lubricated and I rested when I needed it. I took notes on a piece of paper which allowed me to be more present and to see patterns so that I could ask the best questions to advance my students. I had the fluorescent light above my desk(s) turned off to avoid migraine triggers. (We moved desks every three months or so, so I had lots of practice asking every time what I needed from the facilities manager.) After a while we just had a shorthand and laughed about it. I asked my manager(s) to send me emails with reminders and instructions so I could refer back to them. I asked people to lunch when I was in the office. My manager in the beginning believed in me when I did not believe in myself.

I was able to articulate to my manager the why of needing to work from home. Cube land was not conducive to my ability to concentrate. It took so much of my energy to block out the background noise that I was fatigued. Getting one to two days away from the noise increased my productivity. It was a win/win! This all happened because I was able to identify what I needed and communicate the why and frame it as support to get my job done. I did not expect that I would get everything, I worked to be creative and reasonable. It was also important for me in those early days to be at the office for part of the week. I was able to hear how other people approached coaching, ask quick questions so that I could be more efficient and to create community. It was important for me to have the mix.

It's All Connected

The phenomenon of pain is complex and so are the connections that support the movement toward thriving. Thriving is a verb, it is not a destination. So is support. It ebbs and flows. I have days where it is important for me to push myself and do things for myself. Other days I need to be gentle with myself and ask for help or let go of my to-do list. It can be confusing to discern which is better each day especially when depression is part of the equation.

It can also be confusing for others who want to support you. That is why it is so important to have clear communication and to not make assumptions. Sometimes what you may need is acknowledgment of how hard things are. A friend of mine calls it the "poor baby." You may not need or want someone to fix anything or do something for you, instead you want to be seen. Poor baby! It hurts! Sometimes I just want to be told that everything is going to be okay. I do not need to hear how or why. Just that it will be. Other times you may need someone to get something from the top shelf or carry the groceries in. I want to do, what I can, when I can. It is part of thriving for me. I also want to be able to count on people for support when I need it. What do you need?

My mantra when I was in my Whole Systems Design program was, "It's all connected!" Your body is all connected. When you have pain in your knee, it affects everything else. It affects how you walk which affects the rest of your muscular-skeletal systems. How I hold my head affects the tension in my shoulders which effects my lower back which effects . . . you get the idea. Our emotions affect our bodies and are part of our bodies. When you are excited, your breath changes and your blood pumps more. When you are sad, you breathe shallowly, your smile disappears and you slump. And your body affects your emotions. Sitting up, breathing deeply and gently smiling gives your emotions new information. Your thinking impacts your emotions and your body and can impact your willingness to be vulnerable or to ask for support. Your beliefs about your connection with something larger than yourself can impact your thoughts, emotions and body. Meaning can make a sensation more or less painful to experience. It is all connected!

Something else that we deal with is the stigma that chronic pain has in our society. When someone is in chronic pain people may see them as whiners, lazy, incapable, unable to cope, aloof, unpleasant, or angry. Doctors may see them as difficult patients because they do not get better, do not respond the way they are "supposed" to, or they suspect them of drug seeking even when they are not requesting pain medication. We can have internal judgments about our experience as well. We may come up against other people's judgments with friends, family, employers and healthcare practitioners. Pain has so much stigma around it that it can be difficult to ask for support. You may feel unworthy, or selfish, or private.

Living with pain is challenging on many levels. We are wired to avoid pain on many levels including physical, emotional, mental and spiritual. Pain is a universal experience and by its nature is one that we tend to want to run away from. Pain is the signal that something is wrong or dangerous. We go into survival mode. This can be a beneficial reaction. "Get out of this situation!" Adrenaline courses through our bodies and enables us to react. We all have experienced pain on one level or another. We get out of the relationship (or not) or we remove our hand from the hot stove. But when the pain is chronic and does not go away, there are new skills and coping mechanisms that need to be developed in order to move from suffering to thriving.

Actively engaging in life takes energy and focus. Energy and focus may be elusive when you are living with the fatigue and exhaustion of pain. Pacing is what allows you to do what you want to, or need to do without overdoing it. It can be a fine line or razor's edge to balance for people who have chronic pain. Finding the right pace takes patience, awareness and persistence: patience because it takes trial and error to discover a good pace; awareness because optimal pacing changes with many factors that are not static; and persistence because it is over time that you are able develop awareness and listen to your body. The awareness and listening to your body goes beyond what is happening in the moment. Because most chronic pain conditions have a delay in consequences, it is important to see the larger patterns. (This is what we work on in Step One.)

For instance, I can have a rebound effect from bodywork. I might feel fine at the time but later it results in a deep ache and a new turn in the cycle of pain. Or a stretching session that felt fine at the time--meaning I worked slowly and didn't go further than I thought I could handle, but results in spasms the next day or two and a new turn of the cycle of pain. So body awareness is more than just being aware in the moment, it is also about being aware of effects and connections over time. I know for myself I need to change my pacing depending on different variables including my flexibility, my quality of sleep and the plan for the whole day (and sometimes the week). This kind of awareness and effective pacing can be supported emotionally and mentally. If you are in a situation where you feel pushed to do something that you know will hurt you, you may need support to do what you know you need to do. My friends are mostly supportive. They may not know what the edge is for me, but I know that they will support my decision. Occasionally they may even ask if I am sure which gives me permission to honor my own pacing and to take a moment to really check in with myself.

The summer of 2014 I made it a priority to work toward being able to do hikes that got me out in nature. In order to work toward my goal, it was important for me to notice the difference between walking on a level surface and doing elevation changes. A one mile walk on a level surface is different than a 1 mile walk with an elevation change of 800 feet. The effects are different when I walk on a dirt trail compared to cement, rocks or sand. In order to be able to do hikes here in the Northwest, I need to be able to do some elevation change. It is important to me to spend time in nature, enjoy the weather and be with my loved ones. I was able to hike almost every weekend that summer and I was able reach my goal hike which was 8 miles with a 1100 foot elevation gain. It took us six hours to hike it through beautiful terrain. We stopped for lunch at a waterfall and took other rest stops along the way. It was about 5 hours of walking at a comfortable pace. In order to be able to accomplish my goal of hiking, I developed a Thriving with Pain PlanTM. (This is covered in the last section of this book.)

I walked almost every day around my neighborhood, stretched to increase flexibility and continued habits of eating healthy. All of this took active steps. I had to be motivated, to believe that it was possible and to take action. I also had to be patient when I could not walk or didn't follow through. The day after a hike, I was so exhausted that I would not do a walk.

I did more hikes the summer of 2014 and saw more of the beauty around Portland, Oregon than I have in the last decade. This is what I call Thriving! I plan to reintroduce this goal this year. Now that I have spent the past nine months on this book, I need more time hiking!

What Stands in the Way?

I am a very self-reliant person. Asking for support and being seen as not capable was very scary for me. I grew up in a home that made it important that I could take care of myself. My father was very busy with work and my mother was an active alcoholic until I was around 11. (She went through about 4 or 5 years of chronic pain with secondary Glaucoma which eventually led to an eye removal surgery.) I was the youngest but I felt that it was important to take care of myself. I realize that everyone has their own issues about support. Some people are needy and have difficulty doing for themselves, they become too dependent. Some can be too self-reliant and block support and community.

It is a balance that is dynamic from day to day and definitely has changed over my journey. On bad days—when I am in a lot of pain and am exhausted—I need a different kind of support than on good days. It can be difficult to know and then communicate what is needed. It is also scary to be dependent on others. What if they cannot or will not follow through? Fear of abandonment and fear of dependency can get in the way of asking for and accepting help or support. Pride. I have always been proud of my independence! (My parents would probably say stubborn!)

When I was in the early years of grappling with the aftermath of the accident, I accepted support knowing that it was temporary—I was going to heal. The achy shoulder, the sharp pain and weakness in my wrists and hands, the pain in my neck, the migraines, the memory issues, the low back spasms, the sciatica were going to heal. So when I received income replacement from my insurance, I knew it was there to support my healing. I received it gratefully. I allowed myself to rest, get treatment and heal.

But as the pain spread and the fatigue settled in and I

wasn't getting better, my world began to shrink. The fear of not knowing what was wrong began to overshadow my life. "When am I going to get back to my life?" What that really meant was that I was not really in my life. I had put my life on hold. Waiting to get back to my normal. When I finally got to the place of accepting what was happening, I applied for Social Security Disability Insurance. This was a huge step because I was admitting that I could not do what I used to do and I did not have any idea of anything I could do. It was also a humbling experience. I could not focus and concentrate well enough to even answer the questions. I asked a friend to come over and help me to fill in the forms.

When I was having such a difficult time with grieving and adjusting to my new normal, I needed more support. I did not feel like I had much to give. I found out later that I really did have a lot to contribute. Just my presence, my ability to receive with grace, my sense of humor were ways that I contributed to my community. I received without demanding or expecting. This made it easier for people to give.

It is easy to lose sight of our connections when you are living a smaller and smaller life, when what you connected about or did with family and friends is no longer available to you. Grief is a real and necessary process. You may lose the day-to-day contact, your ability to engage in certain pursuits the way you have before, but that does not mean the connections, values and passions are gone.

Pain and fatigue was making doing less possible. I especially had a hard time making plans. I have always been responsible and I do not like making commitments that I cannot keep. I was experiencing a pretty consistent level of pain that I could plan on but it was the flares in fatigue, additional pain and migraines that I could not plan on or around.

As a result, I did not make plans. I finally realized what I was doing-- isolating myself. It was not my friends who turned away from me. It was not even the pain itself that cut me off. It was me. I began to make plans again but I warned people that it was a definite maybe. If they needed a definite yes—buying non-refundable tickets that couldn't be exchanged, then I said "no". If they were okay with my needing to back out at the last moment, then I said "yes". Slowly, overtime, I was able to make those definite maybes into most likely yeses. Making plans actually made me feel better, I had things to look forward to and pace around which improved my mood.

Rhiannon, my partner, put together a great 50th birthday party for me--almost 12 years after the accident. There were probably around 30 plus people that came together to celebrate. I was overwhelmed. They played improvisational games even though some of them were not so excited about that part and they did a no-talent variety talent show (some of them did have talent.) My friends, my community came together to celebrate me. There were many who could not make it. Some people who were there knew me before the accident but many did not. I built a community through connecting, being, communicating, and occasionally doing. But in that evening I was reminded that we are all connected and we impact many. Even in our absence. There were letters from some of my siblings who I rarely see but I know that love and feel connected to me and I to them.

Thriving Lunch

I went to lunch with two women friends who live with Fibromyalgia and other chronic health issues. It was a much-needed session of support and a wonderful illustration of what thriving with chronic pain is all about. If you saw us, we would have looked like any trio of girlfriends getting together for lunch; talking, laughing and sympathizing. But for me, it was a lifeline. I did not have to pretend it was not a bad pain day and that the changes I was doing in my treatment were taking me close to the rabbit hole of pain and depression. Instead, I was able to say how hard it has been lately. That my pain levels have increased as I am changing a protocol that I think will be better in the long run, but right now kind of sucks.

We talked of childhood dogs, the loss of nouns and words, the Neanderthal walk that we do in the morning as our bodies warm up, favorite practitioners and families of origin. This connection is just like any other social connection that increases our quality of life. The thing is, these women understand the world of living with chronic pain. They get it. And they get that wallowing does not serve anyone or anything. Neither does ignoring the reality of living with pain. They also have a sense of humor about the trivialities. It is comforting.

We talked about creativity, projects to make a difference in our communities and how lucky we are that we have great parks around us. Each of us is living our Wow! We have good and bad pain days. We have good and bad emotional days. But we have, each in our own way, taken responsibility for our health. We have searched out proactive protocols including nutrition and alternative practitioners that support our health. We connect with others on a regular basis for support and reach out to others. We follow our passions for creativity, service and purpose in ways that we can. We have come to a place of acceptance so that we have peace in our lives. We are thrivers, one step at a time.

Please share your thriving story and become a part of the thriving community. Go to www.thrivingwithpain.com and share your story and join the community. If you do not feel like a thriver yet and are ready to go from Ow to Wow, take the quiz on the website and keep moving forward through these steps.

Exercise #7—Support Inventory

Community offers support. Support is anything or anyone who makes your life fuller. This can be physical, emotional, social, mental, or spiritual. You can also give support to others. Take an inventory by answering the questions below in your Thriving Journal.

- What is in your life already? (What kind of support do you have in your life right now?)
- Who is in your life? (Who is in your community? Open your mind to the possibility that there are more people than you first can think of. Use the prompt, who else?)
- Do you have pets that bring love and comfort?
- What physical supports do you have (i.e. chair, cane, brace, desks, bed)?
- What supports you to live your life as fully as you do right now?
- Do you have a spiritual community or beliefs?

Exercise #8—Quality of Connections

- What are the quality of your connections?
- Do you feel like you understand what you need?
- Are you able to articulate your experience and your needs?
- What stands in your way of asking for and accepting what you need?
- Do you recognize the gifts that you do have to give?
- How do you support others?

Exercise #9—Physical Support

- What do you need to feel physically supported to thrive?
- Are you more comfortable and supported by being barefoot or wearing shoes?
- Can a brace support you?
- If you have Fibromyalgia doing things overhead can be exhausting.
- Can you ask for help to get something off the shelves in a grocery store?
- Do you have a step ladder to do things around the house?
- Are you willing to use one of the electric carts at the store so you have more energy later?
- As you read these questions, what comes up for you?
- Do you feel ready to ask for support of others or be seen with these supports, or do you feel resistance?
- What is the resistance about?
- Is it more important to you to allow that resistance to get in the way of support?
- Does that resistance take you closer to thriving or suffering?

Exercise #10—Tools for Community

- How do you stay connected?
- What do you want to add to your tool box for connecting? Clear communication? Healthy boundaries?
- I have tools to stay connected; social media, plans, being open and honest, being there for others, asking for what I need, giving what I can. What tools do you have?

Step Four: Engage with Passions, Purpose and Life!

*Let yourself be silently drawn by the stronger pull of
what you really love.*

Rumi

Live with Intention

Thrivers live with intention. An intention to go beyond suffering and survival in order to engage purpose, meaning and to live with passion. For most people this takes time and includes a process of grief. During this process, they make the decision to live. Maybe not the life they had planned, but a new life worth living. Once this decision is made, a lot needs to be done, to learn and to live. They need to find their organizing principles and new expressions. This is the essence of Step Four.

I was in pain, exhausted and depressed. My injuries were not getting better. No matter how much rest or physical therapy I did, I could not do massage without hurting myself. Teaching was not a viable option because of the fluorescent lights which triggered migraines and I could not find words due to the brain fog. Healing was a fulltime job between medical appointments, resting, physical therapy and fatigue. Trying to figure out how to make a living was exhausting, scary and depressing.

When I was in the depths of my fatigue and depression, being passionate about anything felt impossible, much less feeling a sense of purpose and meaning. When I began to explore what brought a spark of interest, humor or joy, I turned toward thriving. These sparks pointed me toward purpose, passion and meaning in my life. I focused my intention on living my life. When you intentionally focus on your wholeness, you pivot toward thriving.

The key skill of Step Four is intention. What is your intention? Sufferers want the pain to stop. Survivors want to not let the pain stop them. Thrivers want to express themselves fully and serve a higher purpose. This is not to say that thrivers would not rather have pain. I, for one, would much rather live pain-free than with chronic pain. Focusing on intention is a skill that can be developed. It is an on-going process. As a thriver, I wake in the morning and I declare my intention for the day. This is what I move toward. Otherwise, the pain and fatigue would be the focus and what I move away from. It is more powerful to move toward something than away from something.

My intention was to enjoy life and to recognize wholeness as I healed. I found meaning in living my theories of healing. I saw the humor in grappling with what had taken me a dozen years to write. How one's wholeness impacts the wholeness of the world. Recognizing wholeness in yourself allows for aligned actions that impact the wholeness of the planet. I was living my personal healing while wanting to connect it to the world; to have meaning and purpose in it. The answer was there in my book, *Path of Heart*. I just had to remember the five doors to explore and remember the connections. My healing journey was my purpose and now I share that in my coaching and now more widely with this book. I have taken my experience and am sharing how I moved from the dark suffering place to a thriving life.

From Caterpillar to Butterfly

The transformation from suffering to thriving is a lot like the transformation of a caterpillar into a butterfly. The caterpillar goes on with its life until it finds itself making a chrysalis in which it turns to goo. I can just imagine the caterpillar thinking, "What the heck, I was doing just fine and now I do not recognize myself at all!" The old way of being and doing fall away. It is the void between who and what you were and who and what you are in your wow. Inside this void, meaning, purpose and passions help to begin to create the new life. You have everything you need as you enter the void to come out the other side as a butterfly. It is not easy or comfortable. It is difficult to see the butterfly in the caterpillar or the goo in the chrysalis, yet it is there. When you focus on the core of you, your being, the goo of you can reorganize into the butterfly. The butterfly emerges because it moves toward becoming itself.

When I was at the end of my rope, a small voice in the back of my head told me it was my fault. I blamed myself. What good was I when I could not do what I used to? What can I do now? Why? I remember the tapes in my mind saying, "if only, I believed in myself more. What did I do to create that car crash? What did I do or think or believe to make this happen?" I had seen many people who had been in car accidents, much worse than mine and they had gotten better. What was wrong with me? There was nothing wrong with me. I was in a chrysalis and breaking down into goo.

One of the things that can get in the way of focusing on wholeness are the changes that happen in our brain due to chronic pain. The limbic system, the emotional center gets hypersensitive and vigilant. Some people blame others and become angry and belligerent. "You would be angry if you were in pain all the time!" Some respond with heightened anxiety and some with depression. The blame whether pointed inward or outward gets in the way of being able to hold an intention. That is why it is so important to remember that the goo has within it the butterfly.

The Grief of Goo

I had just finished my Master of Divinity. It was an Interfaith Divinity program with an emphasis in New Thought. I was surrounded by people who believed that our thoughts create our reality. What does it mean that I am not getting better? But for the life of me, I could not figure out why I had created it. I did not want to be in pain. I had just finished writing my first book, *Path of Heart: Personal and Planetary Healing* when the accident happened. I wanted to get that work out into the world. Instead, I was in the goo and living the theories I had written about. My definition of healing was recognizing the wholeness that already exists. Now I was smack in the middle of brokenness and needing to recognize the wholeness that already existed. The wholeness I needed to recognize was the core of me and my place in the wholeness of the world. This core is like the DNA that allows for the transformation from caterpillar, to goo, to the butterfly.

When I was the gooiest was when I went through the

process of Social Security Disability Insurance (SSDI). I finally admitted that the pain, fatigue and brain fog were making it impossible for me to work. I could no longer be that caterpillar. I finally accepted it and asked for help. I had worked for years to get to the other side, to be able to work but every time I had tried, I could not sustain it. The biggest issue for me was that I could have good days when the brain fog only came in the afternoons and the pain was at a level that I could do things with pacing. Then the bad days would come. I would need to be in bed with the lights out. The brain fog would roll in and I could not track or concentrate. I could not do much of anything. Some bad days I could predict and worked to avoid but others came out of the blue. I could not count on myself much less be responsible to an employer or clients. I was still trying to be the caterpillar while I was goo!

The application process for SSDI was humbling. I could not keep my thoughts together enough to fill out the paperwork. I was frustrated and stressed. Finally, I asked a friend who had been a nurse to help. We spent hours together over a couple of weeks filling out the paperwork and answering questions. This was a friend who had known me only since the accident, yet she was amazed at how much I was affected and how it blocked my abilities. It showed me how well I had hidden my pain and fatigue. Not being able to concentrate or track made the paperwork impossible to do alone. It was difficult to communicate my experience and answer the questions.

The independent physician visit was not fun. It was humiliating. I felt like a suspect sitting in the waiting room. The doctor was there to pass judgment on me and not heal. The issue for me is that I can do things (i.e. I have good range of motion), so on good days I am able to accomplish tasks. I just cannot sustain it. If I overdo, pain and exhaustion increase. The pain and the subsequent fatigue and brain fog are things that the doctor cannot see. Another issue is that it is unpredictable when the pain and fatigue will increase to a disabling level. This is true for many with chronic pain and it is frustrating. I had fought so long because I could do things at times and I did not want to let go of my ability to earn money for my survival and to pursue purpose.

I was turned down for SSDI. This happens in most cases but I was angry. I had gotten to the point of asking for help and accepting what I had been fighting for years—I had raised the white flag. It took me a lot to get to this point and I was told "no". No, you are not really disabled. No, we do not believe you. What!?!?! In the packet they sent me with the rejection was a list of resources, one of them was the state of Oregon's Vocational Rehabilitation Services. "Fine! If you think I am not disabled, you tell me what I can do!" I felt humiliated, angry, scared and out of my depth. I was in complete goo mode!

In the goo, the person you were before is no longer recognizable. There is a time of grief that needs to be honored. The five stages of grief are denial, anger, bargaining, depression and acceptance according to Kübler-Ross model. These stages are not linear but they support letting go of what was and opening to what will be. I spent years in the bargaining working to figure out how I could still be that caterpillar.

It takes time for grief. It cannot be rushed. It takes as long as it takes to turn to goo and to begin to form anew. I am still sad that I cannot do bodywork because I enjoyed my practice. It is a loss. When I do give massages to friends now I am more focused on myself so that I do not hurt myself. This takes away the feeling of selflessness that I used to have. What I do now with coaching changes lives, heals and brings even more of me into my work. My knowledge of how the body works and alternative therapies; my empathy and compassion are now being used in a new way. This change is a win. What goes in the chrysalis, comes out in a new form. When I was finally able to let go and move forward, I had no idea that there would be a butterfly on the other side.

What is Your DNA?

When the caterpillar enters the chrysalis stage it has within it everything it needs to emerge as a butterfly; it is in its DNA so to speak. The expression looks very different from caterpillar to chrysalis to butterfly but it is still the same being, the same DNA. When I went into Vocational Rehabilitation Services to find out what kind of help they could give me, I was smack in the middle of the goo stage. I cried in my intake interview. I felt broken and hopeless. I had already given up. I was no longer the caterpillar but I could not imagine the butterfly. We looked at my abilities, what I was interested in and what I could do now. In a way, we began to look at my core, my DNA.

We each are unique so our expression of our wholeness is different. We each value, are motivated by and are gifted differently. When you are in the goo stage, you can explore these and begin to see what your Wow can look like. It is the process of the chrysalis that allows us to emerge as the butterfly. Purpose, meaning, values, passions and creativity are touchstones that can help you to rediscover your core in this new form.

One of the reasons I liked being a Massage Therapist was that it was physical. I liked working with my hands. It was meditative. I began to explore what I could do that included those things. For example, I began to do projects with wood. I remember when I was a kid going over to a neighbor's house. His father showing us how to work with wood and make skateboards. We used the jigsaw to make the skateboard tops and I remember the smell of saw dust and the feel of sanding down the wood. We attached new rubber wheels. Before that my skateboard had metal wheels. I felt so cool! We got to then use a wood burning tool to write on the top of the skateboard to make it unique. I felt so proud of that skateboard--it rode much quieter than the metal wheels!

I began with small projects and used wood we had milled from a tree that we had to cut down. I made planters, benches and gates. I got to use my hands, my body, my creativity and my intuition. I worked slowly in 5-10 minute increments to start but I got there. It was a great lesson in the power of moving and pacing, and my passions began to leak out. I got excited about doing projects and I felt a sense of accomplishment. I am not a great carpenter. I was working with warped boards sometimes but it was satisfying to see a finished product. The process of creating became a tool in connecting with my passions and a meditative state of flow.

You can look back at your caterpillar self and look at what gave you a sense of purpose and meaning, what your passions and values were. Digging deeper into these can illuminate what is at your core. There are many approaches to this. Following an inquiry of interests, passions, purpose and meaning can help new or mutated passions/interests to emerge. Do you already have a process that you can use for this? If you do, great! Use it! If not, here are some tools that you can use to help get some perspective on yourself and what matters to you. Use these as guides to support your exploration of what is at your core, your DNA. Each of these are deep wells of information that can take you years to understand. At this point, use them as a way to gain perspective so you can see what has meaning, purpose, and value for you so that you can create your thriving life.

- Myers-Briggs Personality assessment information (www.myersbriggs.org) and free place to take abbreviated version: (www.16personalities.com/free-personality-test)
- Jungian Archetypes: Jung, a Psychologist who studied with Freud, put together archetypes that can be interesting to explore as you look more deeply into your own motivations and purpose. You can get more information on this at (en.wikipedia.org/wiki/Jungian) Carolyn Myss has done some work with these more recently and you can get a simplified introduction and test at (www.archetypes.com)
- The Enneagram is another personality and spiritual typing system that is self-reflective. Here is a link to free tests and then more information. www.9types.com and www.enneagraminstitute.com
- *The Artist's Way* is a book by Julia Cameron about harnessing the creative flow. It has a companion workbook.
- *The Life You Were Born To Live: A Guide To Finding Your Life Purpose*, by Dan Millman looks at your life purpose through your birthdate.

I brought myself into the chrysalis which included my skills, knowledge and values. I had short term memory issues and physical limitations so the outward expression would be different. As I went through a number of processes, exercises and inventories to identify my abilities, as well as my interests and what was available in the market place, the butterfly began to take shape.

I love to work with people and to make a difference. I am empathetic and compassionate. I value healing as I define it; recognizing wholeness that already exists. Love, humor, balance, learning, fun and growth are some of my core values.

After deep diving, I decided that if I could work, I wanted to be a coach. Many people over the years have said I would make a great therapist but I had decided long ago that I didn't want to deal with that kind of responsibility. A coach works in partnership with the client to deal with what is, what they want, what it will take to move forward, make action plans and hold the client accountable while supporting them through the barriers and challenges that arise. I see therapists as an expert that helps guide the client/patient through developmental issues, delving into the past and dealing with issues and possibly supporting people through emotionally difficult times such as grief, change, or growth. I have personally benefited from therapy off and on in my life and believe that it is a great process. I am clear it is not in my DNA, but coaching is.

So I looked into becoming a coach and how to get trained. I did research about what it would take to move forward. I was nervous about whether I could do it given my concentration issues. As I was surfing the internet, I found a job posting for a Success Coach with a company that worked with universities to retain students and increase graduation rates. I was shocked. I believe in life long learning and the value of education. It was right there in front of me and I thought it might be too good to be true. I called Vocational Rehabilitation to see what I could do to prepare myself for the interview, if I got one, and to find out how they could support me moving forward. I got the interview, which turned out to be two interviews and I got the job. It was a great fit! I began the journey of being employed as a coach. The goo was definitely beginning to take a shape.

Moving Toward—Not Away From

I have been to the place of suffering and blame. I know the depth of major depression and the experience of waving the white flag and not getting support I thought I needed. I have slowly over time rediscovered my passions and meaning after grieving the loss of what had been before. I did not go head long into meaning, renewed passions and purpose. It was a process. First, I had to discern what I could and could not do. I had to let go of and grieve what I lost. Then I had to explore meaning, purpose and my passions in this new life. When I could begin to explore what brought a spark of interest, humor or joy, I began to thrive. This came in the form of getting a dog, staying connected to friends, meditating, building things, writing, coloring and enjoying books and movies.

Small Things and Small Steps

It really is the small stuff that make the biggest difference. Small enjoyments like the feel of sunshine, the sound of the waves, the smell of a forest, the happy wagging tail of your dog, or the sound of bird song can help to dispel suffering. I was blessed to live in the country when I was healing from my accident. Breathing in the air in the morning while I had my first cup of tea on our porch and looking at the greenery and wildlife soothed my soul. Finding meaning and purpose in my new life was difficult. I looked at my past passions to find the kernels to bring forward. I found new ways for them to be expressed. I discovered new passions. Even today my limbic system can get triggered, however these small things that heal my limbic system are incredibly powerful.

Going from Ow to Wow is not something that can be done

with big steps. It is made up of small steps that change your perspective from 'moving away from pain' to 'moving toward thriving'. It is when you ignite your willingness to observe wonder in yourself, others and the world that you can begin to answer these questions for yourself—what is it all about? What is important to me? What do I value? What is my intention?

With every road block or detour in life comes an opportunity. What are the gifts? It takes time to discern. Without this journey into chronic pain, I might still be a massage therapist and teacher. Instead, I have a mission to bring hope, tools and advocacy to the hundreds of millions who live with chronic pain. I love supporting people to live their Wow and thrive. The obstacles and barriers that create the Ow are part of the Wow. Without these, the butterfly would never have strong enough wings to fly. This is my butterfly.

Day by day we live our lives. We make small but important decisions that overtime become our habits. It may be that you wake up one day to find that your life has shrunk because of all the things you no longer do. Your life is almost unrecognizable. This can also work the other way. Small steps taken everyday can take you to a new life, one that you did not think possible.

Our thoughts and words have power--the power to shape our perceptions, to show us our wholeness or to point us toward suffering. I treasure my experience of fire-walking because I learned the power of intention and focus, and the power of self-doubt. I learned that the seemingly impossible is possible with a community encouraging you. (We covered community and support in Step Three.) Now I can face my fears and step across the fire by staying focused on what is important: the intention of the destination. It is not the destination itself that is important but the focus of the intention. These lessons have stayed with me through the years and I can pull on this knowing when I can face what seems impossible because of my fears. I remember that I can walk across fire. Getting to the other side of the fire is not the point, it is the how; the intention. I can do anything with the power of intention. Look ahead to what is important and stay present in the moment. Surround yourself with a supportive community who can hold the intention with you. It is both intention and presence. Love yourself, live with intention and life is good!

The Purpose of Wow!

A life of Wow is a life of purpose. It is a life Willingly Observing Wonder! You connect to the wonders around you and notice awe. This connects you to something greater than yourself. Meaning and purpose infuses your life by connecting you to something larger. You embrace your gifts through your interests, passions and creativity. It is a life of both/and/plus. You take care of yourself and at the same time you move beyond yourself. Your gift is who you are and how you are in the world. In expressing your gifts, you can be focused on the intention of the destination. You can ignore the fire under your feet and walk unscathed toward your destination. You are using the highest form of distraction-- self-transcendence.

We are unique and therefore our gifts are unique. Your Wow is a clear expression of your wholeness. Sometimes my wholeness is more gracefully expressed than others. When you are "Willingly Observing Wonder", you are bringing WOW to the forefront. Wonder in the world around you, yourself and others. It is not always pretty; it does not always appear to be perfect. It is in resilience and persistence that thriving and WOW are expressed.

What we do and how we do it impacts the world. We may never know exactly how we make it. I remember vividly in my younger years when I was dealing with depression, a woman walked by and smiled at me. I had been swirling around in despair and that smile lit up my heart. I felt the despair lighten and a sense of connection pulling me out of the darkness. She did not know that her smile helped me to pull out of a horrible place and helped me to go on. Decades later, I still remember it! I believe this is true in the absence as well. If we refuse to do what is ours to do, no one else can. Our gift is not in the world if we do not bring it. The world is less whole without our gift!

The Role of Creativity

When you are having a bad pain day or you are tired of being sick and tired, it can be difficult to connect with something larger. Creativity is a way to connect. As I shed my old self, my professional pursuits, and lost most of my energy, I had to come into myself and see what I had to live for. Life itself is precious. Any day above ground is a good day. Engaging in creativity, connecting, meditating and pleasant activities such as coloring, building a planter, playing with our dog(s) are all ways to connect with a life larger than self. Every morning I have my cereal and tea and my dogs get up on my lap and we have our morning snuggle. Something this simple can be the ground for Wow.

I am not an artist, although I live with one. Creativity is not just for artists. It is a mind space that allows for touching the super conscious, as Jung called it. For me, this space is expansive, healing, connecting and relaxing. It is like touching infinity. Some call it flow. You do not need to be Michelangelo to connect with flow. It is a sense of connecting with something larger than you and expanding expression through creativity.

When I began to build projects around the house, I did

not do so with this in mind. I just knew that I needed to do something to get out of my head and to distract me from what I was no longer able to do. What I found is the power of following the little signs of interest, creativity and purpose. The small steps and small acts moved me forward to the next step, the next small act until an 'aha' moment happened. The 'aha' was that with purpose and meaning I could live a life larger than myself even while living with pain.

When you live with pain and you are a survivor, your life is not necessarily driven by the pain like a sufferer's is but it is still organized around it. Being a survivor means that the thing (pain) that you are surviving has an impact on your identity and how you organize your life. You begin to identify with the pain and it runs you, rather than you running your life. When I realized that I needed something larger than myself to organize my life around, I began the path of thriving. When I work with clients, I step outside of myself and my experience. I listen from a deep place; reflect back that wisdom; explore with curiosity; share resources and hold accountability with compassion. I am able to do this, in part, because I have been there. I have compassion for my clients and the process of healing.

This process was born out of my life experience with chronic pain, my gifts, knowledge and skills. I approach life from the perspective of interconnections and creativity that I learned in my Graduate Program in Whole Systems Design including heart/mind/body/spirit connections that I explored deeper in my massage therapy practice. In my Master's project for Whole Systems Design, I defined healing as, "recognizing wholeness that already exists." This definition holds within it the perspective of wholeness and not fixing something broken. In one of my first workshops on Personal and Planetary Healing—Making the Connections, a participant who worked in the medical field expressed a sense of relief at my definition. Trying to fix something that is broken takes effort and has a sense of responsibility where as recognizing wholeness is relaxing into a knowing. I began that inquiry because of the burnout I saw in social movements. To fix is to fight against; to recognize is to allow what already is and allow it to blossom.

Being a thriver moves beyond seeing the brokenness. You focus on the Wow (wholeness) and not the Ow (brokenness). "Sure, easy for you to say!", you may be thinking. But the truth is, it was not easy for me. Even now, I have to consciously hone my intention to put the wholeness in the forefront. I had written the book on healing, on recognizing wholeness and now I practice it. I have not perfected it. But through these steps, I found my way back to my whole self, found strength and courage I did not know I possessed, and am now supporting others to get their lives back more quickly and with less struggle.

I have heard people in my support groups say that pain had hollowed them out. When pain comes in and steals all that was true, it takes time to fill yourself back up. There is a time to rebuild, to find the gifts of the hollowing, to find the seeds of passion, purpose and/or service. Getting into a creative activity is a positive step toward thriving. When I color, do collages, create and do ceremonies and rituals, build and garden, I feel bigger when I am doing it. I feel I am in the flow; my attention and intention are engaged in creation—not on my pain.

When your life is shadowed by pain there needs to be organizing principles and values that pull you forward and not just away from pain. I was working with a healthcare team. I kept waiting to be better enough to be able to do massage again. I was doing my healing work; receiving massage, physical therapy, resting, stretching etc. but I never got to that point. As

I grieved the loss of my professional dreams, I was adrift. Yet I had my faith, my partner, my values, and creativity supported me to stay focused on the good.

Being creative doesn't mean you have to be a master artist. Engaging the non-linear creative side of your brain can decrease stress and take you to that more expansive mind space. Creativity is one of the abilities we have as humans. When you are in pain, it can be difficult to engage in anything positive. That is why you start where you are and take small steps. Adult coloring books are very popular and are a great way to engage creativity. One of my friends mentioned that she always takes a set of pens and a small coloring book with her.

I built things when I was recovering. It took me quite a while since I could only work for five to fifteen minutes at a time but slowly creating planters, pergolas, and a shed gave me great satisfaction. They were not wonderful works of art. Over time I got better at creating things that did not fall down. But the process was important. I learned new skills and I had something concrete at the end of my exertion. It was okay if I cried out in pain (there was no one there to get startled unlike my clients on the massage table). Last year I created a workbench for Rhiannon to start her glass torch work studio so she could create glass beads. My creativity served her creativity. I would never had guessed that my basic carpentry work would result in my having jewelry!

Every Day is a New Day!

I believe we all have these choices in every moment no matter the circumstances which we find ourselves. So how do I make that choice? Can it get easier? Yes, it is like a muscle that needs to be developed and exercised. Every time I can be 'at cause', the more I am able to take charge of my life. Every time I am 'at effect' (I react), I lose power. Two powerful tools in making this happen are proactivity and intention.

- First, know that I want to choose; clarity of intention and confidence that I can choose.
- I want to live a full life that brings joy, healing, laughter and meaning. {Check}
- I want to live responsibly knowing that I am responsible for my reactions. {Check}
- Second, I have to make choices that reflect these intentions and take action.
- I do my stretches, take my medications, and meditate. {Check}
- I call a friend and make a date to go to tea or just chat on the phone making sure laughter and connection are at the center of the interaction. {Check}
- Third, I live in the present with an understanding that what is, is what will be.
- What I choose today in this moment will move me closer to my desired way of being or will pull me away from it. {Check}
- I take a walk and play with my dogs. I choose healthy habits that I know are good for me. {Check}

But still, those nagging thoughts of, "It's not fair!" and "I don't deserve this pain!" creep in. I can feel the cloud of depression and overwhelm in the corner of the room and my mind. I choose to breathe and remember that I am not alone, that the separation is just an illusion. I am connected and I can shine a light into the cloud and know that it doesn't have control over me.

The more times I practice, the easier it becomes. It is not 100%. That is why I know I am not a saint, yet! I have choice and that choice supports me to feel more alive, more joy, more blessed and to laugh more. I can also choose to wallow. There are times, days that I do. Not very often but when I choose to, I go for it! Yell, cry, roll into a ball. IT ISN'T FAIR!!!!! Well what is fair? Things happen. What is, just is. This is hard for me to understand but when I think of the alternative, it would mean that I did something to deserve my pain, to deserve losing my massage practice, etc. On a bad day I can go on and on about what I have lost, what I have suffered. I long for my life as a caterpillar. . . silly butterfly!

The Gifts of WOW

On most days I remember that there are gifts with each of those losses; that I could never have become a thriver if I did not have the obstacles and barriers to overcome. Being a thriver has allowed me to discover my resilience, persistence, courage and compassion (especially for myself). One of the most powerful tools that I have discovered is WOW. When you are experiencing pain it is easy to focus on that and allow your awareness to reduce to only the pain. The pain is like a hyperactive, loud five-year-old that is working hard to get your attention. "Hey, look at me! Look at the drawing I made on the wall! Oops, there goes my blueberry juice on the carpet and furniture!" In the midst of this, WOW (Willingly Observing Wonder) allows you to breathe. Wonder is awe, gratitude and love all rolled into one. When you can focus your will on observing wonder in your life, pain no longer is the center of attention. My journey from ow to WOW has led me to my new vocation of working with others who have chronic pain, in a new way. I worked with many people with chronic pain as a massage therapist. Now that I know from my own experience what it can mean to live with pain, I come to this work with a new perspective.

WOW does not mean ignoring the five-year-old (pain), it means opening up to wonder. Marveling at the wonders of nature, of my community, of the goodness in the world, of the quiet place of peace inside that can be touched through mindfulness and meditation. Breathing in the knowledge of the non-pain in my body.

My experience gives me credibility. My experience has turned my theories of healing into practice. I also know that everyone is different. I learned that quite literally through my decade of massage practice and from my partner. She has chronic pain and she is almost always the opposite in what works and what does not even though we have similar diagnoses. There is no cookie cutter approach that works for everyone. Each massage I gave responded to the body on the table. No two were alike, even on the same person.

Now I am able to know that I can choose to stay in suffering, be stoic, be a survivor or thrive at anytime. Each time I make a choice that brings me closer to recognizing wholeness and willingly observing wonder, the closer I am to being able to make the next choice more easily. The muscle of thriving is developed and new neuropath ways are forged. Thriving takes intention, time, choice and persistence.

The gifts of thriving are beyond measure. I can support others because of what I have been through. I have a sense of accomplishment and joy with the small things in life. My pain has diminished as I have become more of a thriver. Thriving can interrupt the pain cycle. It is hopeful! When in doubt pivot to thriving. Choose one point on the Thriving cycle and dive into Thriving.

Exercise #11—Thriving Focus

Community, creativity, beauty, nature, building something, playing, leading, performing, pleasure are ways for me to focus on thriving.

- What ways do you to focus on thriving?
- What instills a feeling of awe in you?

Exercise #12—Explore the Small Things

What has meaning for you? What are you interested in? What feels purposeful? Everyone is different. Fashion, beauty, animals, music, social change, politics, dance, gardening, history, philosophy, sports, food, or . . . are all possible arenas that can give you direction for Step Four.

Exercise #13—Acknowledge Your Losses

What have you lost due to the pain?

Acknowledge them: Once you have written the list create a ritual to let them go. One way to do this is a burning bowl (or you can use a fire place.) Take some time to read each thing that you have lost and then burn each one separately letting go as the fire takes the words. You can do this alone or with someone from your community who can witness this with you. By letting them go you can begin to see what comes next.

Exercise #14—Engage

Use the following questions as prompts in your journal.

- Do you engage in any creative pursuits?
- Are you involved with anything larger than yourself?
- What stops you, if you are not engaged?
- Do you engage in any creative pursuits?
- What do I have to give?
- What is my purpose?
- What meaning can I find in my life? For many having a spiritual faith brings purpose.

Exercise #15—Interest and Values

Take one of your interests or values and write for 10 minutes without stopping, why you like it. You can start by filling in the sentence and then use the sentence anytime you get stuck. If you cannot write that long, talk into a recording device. Let the words flow and do not edit yourself.

- "I like _____ because ..."
- Come back to it another time and write about how you have expressed these interests and values in your life before.
- "When I _____ before I ..."

Exercise #16—Core Values

Use the following questions as prompts in your journal.

- What are your top five core values?
- What interests you most?
- For this exercise list the things that you are/were interested in even if you do not see how you can engage with them.
- What are you passionate about or were?
- Do you like to create or engage with creativity?
- What do you find meaningful?
- What is your intention for your life?
- What makes you smile?
- What do you highly value?
- What is your vision for your new life?

Exercise #17—Get Creative or Destructive!

A coloring book with a set of pencils or crayons, tissue paper and a glass candle, humming a song, knitting, finger/toe/ or nose painting, or origami.

That creative spark allows entry into the super-conscious and stress relief. Maybe creativity is too much for you right now. Maybe destruction would help. Get some plates and smash them, take down a wall, or split firewood.

Step Five: Live Mindfully and Thrive!

God, Grant me the Serenity to accept the things I cannot change.
Courage to change the things I can, and
The wisdom to know the difference.
The Serenity Prayer

I have been pondering the words of the Serenity Prayer lately. As I reflect on my work with chronic pain, I realize that these words hold a key to thriving. Truly, whatever challenges, obstacles and barriers you face, this type of acceptance points the way. We need courage to take powerful actions that change what we can. We need wisdom to know what powerful actions are and when we cannot change something. We need the ability to accept and not be resigned when we cannot change something. This acceptance is powerful because it is based in the present moment and gives a ground for being. Resignation is deflating because it is based in the past and the future, "It has and always will be this way!"

Acceptance of what is, allows for change. Courage to act allows for movement. Wisdom to know the difference gives you insight into leverage points that can make the difference in the quality of life. It is a process.

Acceptance versus Resignation

It is easy to confuse acceptance and resignation. 'The doctors say I will never walk again'; 'The doctors say I will always have this pain and I just need to live with it'; 'I will never have friends again because who wants to be around me.' Resignation puts up a barrier to change. Energy is dissipated and flattened. Depression creeps in. Hope flees. You do what is necessary but there is no spark. It truly takes courage to act in the face of acceptance of what is and hope that things may change. Finding leverage points that give you a better chance for success are important. (We will cover more in the Thriving with Pain Plan section.) Living in the present and on life's terms is a skill and an attitude that can be learned. No matter where you start it is possible. In this way of living, there is power, serenity, and wisdom.

"You are going to have to learn to live with your pain and accept it," doctors tell their patients when they do not have any physical treatment options left. But how are you going to learn? A referral to a therapist or psychologist can make you think the doctor does not believe you, or s/he thinks it is all in your head. Pain is a biological, psychological and social phenomenon. The brain is part of the pain experience and literally is altered with years of continued pain. If you are lucky you are referred to someone who understands chronic pain. There are psychological therapies that can help you to reduce pain and re-wire your brain. It does not mean it is not real or that you are making it up in your head.

Acceptance is a process and going through the preceding four steps aids your discernment. Becoming an expert on yourself, working with treatments that aid you to change what you can and connecting with community all help you to develop the skills, tools, and attitudes to make changes and heal. When you pivot to what is important to you; a positive focus of meaning and purpose, you are able to live with intention.

When you live in reaction to your circumstances, you have no power. When you bring your center into yourself, you begin to own your power through your reactions—or really your response. Reactions are like reflexes—no thought, no conscious choice. Response comes from a place of choice. Reflexes are necessary but when they overtake everything, you live in the Ow; afraid of everything and at the mercy of your circumstances. Living your life with the stress response triggered most of the time increases pain and creates an inability to deal and heal. When you are able to increase the opposite, the parasympathetic nervous system which helps with rest and digest, you are able to heal and thrive.

Life on Life's Terms

Learning to accept life on life's terms is incredibly powerful. Especially for those of us with chronic pain. Non-acceptance is a form of resistance. You may have heard the saying, that which you resist, persists. It is a fundamental law of systems theory. When you are dealing with a system that is self maintaining, it has feedback loops that will push back. When you focus on resisting the pain, it persists. When you focus on allowing without judgment, pain tends to diminish. Acting from a place of resistance also increases stress which adds to your already overloaded body, which typically increases pain. Let me be very clear about something. Acceptance and resignation are very different. Acceptance is active and empowering. It is being in the moment and allowing life to unfold as it is. Resignation is passive and depressing. When you are resigned, you may exist but you are not fully present in your life and you are not thriving. It is the difference between suffering and thriving. It is a process of discernment between what you can influence and what is beyond your influence. Accepting what you do not have influence over in the moment and acting to effect what you can.

This is why this Step of Acceptance is last in these five steps. In order to truly accept and not just be resigned, you need to develop the courage to make the changes that you can and have the wisdom to know what cannot be changed. You make changes that allow you to live and not just exist. You accept what you cannot change and thrive. Each moment offers you new information. What was not able to be changed in the past, may change now or in the future. (The only constant in life is change.) The skill of awareness supports the process of discernment which is ongoing. This is what Step One supports. Awareness and discernment aid in the process of acceptance. Exploring your treatment options and taking action is what Step Two is all about. Research regarding pain and its treatment may give you tools to change things down the road.

Let me tell you a secret: doctors do not know everything. They tell patients every day what they think is happening (diagnosis) and will happen (prognosis). We go to them to figure out what to do about it (treatment). They have years of knowledge about the body and if they keep up with research in their area of expertise, they may know things that you cannot access on your own. They understand what science and medicine knows about the body and mind. Yet still doctors' knowledge is not always right. I have known people who have lived decades beyond their life expectancy given their prognosis; people who walked again after being told they would not; and people who were declared to be in perfect health who die that very night.

We know that pain happens in the brain. It was not that

long ago that it was believed that nerve pathways were static. Now we know that there is the ability for them to change, something called neuro-plasticity. Living in the future of "if only" or "when" does not allow you to be present now, where you can thrive, where your true power lives. Hope does. Acceptance does. Living life on life's terms means you accept that stuff happens, pain happens and that you can see the wondrousness of life. Focus on wholeness and not brokenness to bring an awareness to life's wonder! What you focus on is brought more into focus. If you focus on your pain and catastrophize about all that it means, can mean and will mean, then you ramp up your nervous system to give you more pain signals. If you focus on wonder, then you breathe deeper, see possibilities, and know wholeness. This is not a pie in the sky, 'Pollyanna' approach. It is a realistic, practical approach that allows for your wholeness to unfold.

You have a choice everyday, in every moment. Focus on the light—what is whole, or focus on the dark—what seems broken. Focusing on wholeness and wonder is a habit that can be developed. The more you focus on the dark, the more you live in the dark. The dark is inhabited by depression, fear, anxiety, and anger. The more you focus on the light, the more you live in the light. The light is inhabited by compassion, kindness, gratitude, love, and connection.

I have lived with depression most of my life. I understand the seduction of the dark; how the black hole can suck one in. I work in my life to focus on wholeness. This was how the definition of healing evolved—recognizing wholeness that already exists. It is not about making something happen. Wholeness is. This was particularly challenging when chronic pain became a reality for me. I took my theory of healing into practice. It is not easy but it is so much better than the alternative. The alternative is to have the brokenness take center stage and have it be the focus of life. When pain is at the center, I contract. Contract physically to protect myself from more pain; contract emotionally to protect myself from more suffering; and contract socially to protect myself from the stigma of pain and fatigue. When I focus on wholeness, I expand to embrace all of life. I focus on the wonder.

It is the How that Creates the What

Pacing is one of the skills that was covered in Step Two. It is an important skill and yet it can become a tool for contraction as well, if it becomes rigid. When you accept what is at the moment, then you have the opportunity to make choices that will increase your pain and your quality of life. (What?, you might say.) Yes, there are times when not pacing is the choice that will increase your quality of life, when you are able to accept the consequences. You may choose to go to your granddaughter's birthday party even though you know it will likely trigger more pain. You have your self-care and pain management skills but you know you will have more pain. Do you do it anyway? What is most important to you? Where are your values? If part of your purpose is being connected to your granddaughter, then you may decide to go. When you are experiencing pain, you can smile knowing it was worth it. That is accepting what is and thriving!

I normally am a great pacer. I take breaks, I plan out big events so that I do not overdo and I allow for recovery time. When I went to the European Pain Congress of EFIC in Vienna in 2015, I chose to go all three days so that I could soak up the experience and get as much information as I could. It was an amazing experience. Besides going to the wrong place the night before when I went to do an early registration, everything went off without a hitch. I navigated the public transit system to get to the conference from the apartment that we had found. When I arrived I found out that there were 4000 people at the Congress and about 3000 of those were doctors. I was excited and nervous! Luckily the official language was English so I could understand most of what was being said. The program was a book, quite literally. It was filled with short descriptions of all the workshops that were being offered. It was huge!

In the area where there were booths, they had everything from new devices, to publishers, to Associations, to products, to a patients' organization. Row upon row. It was a bit overwhelming. They even had a "machine of pain" that was there to have doctors experience neuropathic pain. You put your hand into a large box through a dark cloth. Electrodes were then placed on the skin of your arm and hand by the 'man behind the curtain'. You did not know what he was doing. You would feel a sensation and you had to tell him when you felt discomfort. He had you explain what the pain felt like. This put the 'receiver' into the position of 'patient'. When I put my arm in the machine, I experienced shooting pains that went up my hand up to my shoulder that then created painful spasms. I felt a burning sensation that felt like someone had placed a hot iron on my skin. I felt prickling up and down my arm like intense sticking with pins and needles that made me want to jump out of my skin. I also experience stabbing sensations up and down my arm. I watched others for a while and really appreciated that this 'black box of pain' was going to medical schools to teach the new generation of doctors what various neuropathic pain feels like instead of relying on only the technical words on a page. Of course, a few minutes of these sensations is nothing compared to living with it day-to-day but it seems like a start for developing some empathy again. The pain in my arm and shoulder was much increased during the rest of the day due to my nerves being stimulated!

The conference center, like many in the world, had cement floors covered by thin carpet. I had already spent a week in Paris where I walked a lot. My legs ached and felt heavier than they had in years but I made a conscious choice to go to workshops. I felt that the information would provide benefits that outweighed the short-term increase in pain. I stood and stretched on the side or in the back of the room. In two presentations I laid on the floor. Because I was being purposeful, I was able to accept the pain and not dwell on it. I also took a hot bath in the evening which made a huge difference. I knew that the pain was increased because I chose not to pace like I would at home, but this was an opportunity of a life-time! I did not want to contract or shrink and miss the opportunity. Even taking a trip to Europe was outside my comfort-zone. But now I can truly say I will always have Paris.

The Intention of Wow

Power is important to understand what is in your influence and what is not . . . in the moment. When you are a sufferer, you do not feel powerful—you feel victimized by the pain. You are affected by the pain but you do not have much power to effect the pain. As a survivor, you have power to overcome the pain but your identity is organized around the pain—you live in spite of the pain. As a thriver, you have the power to affect and accept the pain and to live a whole life regardless of the pain.

How you do what you do creates the environment for what you create. I went into the Vienna Congress with a plan. I followed through with self-care and pain management techniques. I went in excited and focused on the possibilities. I learned, I connected, I experienced, and I gained confidence. What I created was a life-long memory of wonder.

I could have easily focused on my pain and the brokenness. The chairs were all too tall. My back was never supported. I had to walk from one end to the other of this very large conference center across hard cement floors which irritated my low back and made my legs feel more and more achy and heavy. There was a presentation that I had to sit on the floor without any support because it was so packed. No one offered me a chair or the wall. Did they not know I was in pain? I did not know anyone there, why were they not trying to get to know me?

Instead, I marveled that so many from all over Europe and some from other parts of the world were coming together to look at the phenomenon of pain and how to treat it. I listened, took notes, and gained an appreciation of the amount of information that doctors are inundated with if they try and stay current. Hundreds, (if not a thousand), of research papers were presented in the poster sessions alone. Experts from every stripe were there to share what they had been studying, all with implications for treating pain. I got up and asked a question in one of the sessions. I connected with the patient organization who pointed me toward the World Institute of Pain. I connected with them and they in turn connected me with the editor of *Pain Pathways* magazine. Nine months later, in the Spring 2016 issue, my article on Ow to Wow appeared in their Reflections section. This "what" came from my "how" of wonder and power.

Mindfulness: The Skill of Acceptance

Mindfulness is a skill. A skill of attention and non-judgment that can create serenity. It is in vogue these days, which is great. There are classes that you can take but really it is something that can be practiced at anytime, anywhere. It is being present in your experience, in your life. Mindfulness is being here, now. It is being in the moment fully without judgments about what should or should not be. Instead, noticing what is.

Mindfulness allows you to notice what is happening. Often I hear that people cannot meditate because they cannot get their mind to quiet or that they cannot sit still. Mindfulness and many meditations are not about making the mind quiet. It is about the process of noticing. Noticing the mind as it races, as tangents are taken, as problems run across the mind and then, without judging, gently bringing your focus on the present moment. If in the present moment your thoughts are filled with the future or the past, you notice that in the present. You do not focus on your worries or plans about the future, nor the regrets or grievances of the past but you notice what it is like to be fully aware in the present of these thoughts and feelings. By witnessing your thoughts, your sensations, your breath, and your actions you accomplish two ends. You become more present, more alive in the moment and you effect the ground of your experience. Being witnessed has an effect, even if you are your own witness.

Studies have shown that meditation and especially mindfulness effect the stress response and decrease pain. The body scan is a great example. This has been done in stress management programs around the United States with great success. It is noticing sensations in your body as you are in a comfortable relaxed position without falling asleep. As you notice and witness, you stay focused on the sensation, turn down the volume on judging what the sensation might mean, and allow it to be without attempting to change anything. This is a skill and it has an effect on your nervous system. Over time, people who have been in these programs have experienced less stress and pain. It shows up in better blood pressure, more steady blood glucose, lower cholesterol, and more activity. It is a simple, effective way to practice and get an idea of what mindfulness is all about. Go to *www.thrivingwithpain.com* and sign up for a free membership and then go to downloads under Resource menu to download a body scan recording. If you are not online, you can use the words in the appendix and record it for yourself.

In Step Two we talked about mindfulness meditation as a treatment option. So why bring it up here again? Mindfulness as a skill of perspective is essential to Step Five—Live Mindfully and Thrive! The mindful perspective witnesses your experience and watches your judgments, desires, and pain non-judgmentally. Paradoxically, this perspective that stands apart also encompasses all of you. This is your sacred witness. A part of you that can hold you with compassion within a context of a larger perspective. This is what I mean by the ground of your experience. With the skill of mindfulness, you are able to shift the context of your experience from an out of control, reactive context to a compassionate, peaceful context. When you change the ground of your experience, you change your inner environment. You can be in a stressful or increased pain environment without it overwhelming you. Mindfulness is a great way to change your environment. This is how you can change something that may have felt out of your control before. "I can't help how I feel!" The truth is that our thoughts and our feelings are something that we can influence by attending to them without judgment, by being mindful. In my experience it is more effective to notice than to actively fight. It is easier to place positive thoughts and attitudes in focus than it is to fight against negative ones. This is exactly what mindfulness does.

Thriving mindfully is a way of life that accepts what is and allows you to live fully. It is not about perfection or always being up and positive. It is not about being pain-free. If you have an expectation of pain relief, you lose the benefits of presence because you are in the future or are judging that it is not working. It is about compassionate self-awareness, empowered actions, supportive community, passionate purpose, and accepting life on life's terms. Throw in some laughter and creativity and you are a Thriver living your Wow!

Thriving is a state of being. I have days, hours, moments when I feel victimized by my body and my circumstances. I get angry, sad, and even depressed. I get reactive, I forget to be pro-active. Yet I am still a thriver. Why? Because I forgive myself, I have compassion and remember I am human. I discover actions and tools that support me to feel empowered again. I am part of a community that I can reach out to instead of beating myself up. I turn on some music, grab a coloring book, talk with a client and get back in touch with what is meaningful. I breathe and get in touch with my sacred witness, that part of me that notices my mindfulness. In other words, I persist. I thrive and so can you!

Living in your body is the best place to really experience your life but pain can make you want to be anywhere but your body. The experience of Ow makes it more difficult to be present in the moment. Each moment gives you access to being alive but if you do not take it, you miss out on feeling alive.

Being present in your body is difficult for many in our world today. It is unpleasant to be present when anger, fear, shame, and despair are what you are experiencing. Through experiencing these emotions, you get to the core of aliveness.

We live in a world of distractions—phones, television, news, past, and the future. These distractions pull us from being present with our lives. It seems easier to not feel, to be numb than to deal with the truth of life. Aliveness is available in each moment, through each breath. Yet it can be uncomfortable or down right painful to touch that aliveness and so many of us actively distract.

What I have found on the other side of this presence is the Wow! If you can allow yourself to be present with yourself, your pain, your experience, you can find a sense of peace and wonder. You can find yourself. When pain happens, it is natural to want to get away from it but staying present without judgment can bring peace and space to make conscious choices instead of living in reaction.

Mindfulness allows for this presence. Being aware, not judging, and accepting what is in the moment are the keys to mindfulness. In this state, if you can stay there when uncomfortable thoughts, feelings, and sensations occur, you can find the power of choice. The conditioning of fear, of avoidance, of judgment can be set aside and life can be met on life's terms.

Laughter

Laughter is the best medicine. It is true but it can sound trite. But finding humor through the pain is powerful. It can be another way to shake loose any old attitudes and thought patterns because it makes fun of that which is painful. I am what I call a "SEU" a Self Entertaining Unit. I find the humor in almost everything.

Having a sense of humor when dealing with life's struggles is a must. I can tell when people have a good sense of humor, they laugh at my jokes! But beyond that, being able to see life with all its twists and turns and quirks and still be able to laugh is the epitome of a good sense of humor. So being a little twisted helps!

Sometimes it can be short interactions that can tickle me. The other night I went to the movies at the Academy Theater in the Montavilla area near my house. I decided to splurge and get some popcorn. I know, not the best thing for me. The corn was probably GMO, it is popped in oil, (my dentist told me popcorn is the #1 reason for cracked teeth) . . . but I decided to do it anyway. The guy serving me asked if I wanted butter. Like I said, I was splurging so I said yes! Then immediately wondered if it was "butter" or some chemical filled substitute.

I asked, "Is it real butter?"

"No," he replied.

I decided I shouldn't have it either way; the question gave me a chance to make a healthier choice and so I declined— "the butter."

As he handed me the popcorn, with a very earnest look he said, "Yeah, we don't use real butter because we want to keep our popcorn vegan."

This cracked me up. I do not know if this would happen somewhere else, but it felt like one of those 'only in Portland' moments. (Check out *Portlandia* for some chuckles and context.) Where else would a movie theater be making sure their popcorn stays vegan!

Things like this happen all the time. Small things that happen around me that crack me up. Maybe it comes from my mom. She allowed us to have fun at her expense and was someone who could laugh at herself. She had a head tremor through out my whole life. It always looked like she was shaking her head no. I think it started around the time I was born or soon thereafter. (At least this is what she told me, like it was my fault.) She was a bit self-conscious about it when she went out in public.

At home we had some fun with it. I remember one time she was on the phone and I wanted to go over to a neighbor's. So I asked her if she minded if I went to my friend's house. She of course shook her head no and I was off, licitly-split, before she could realize that she had given me permission to go! See this is part of how I got a little twisted, it was always better to phrase the question so that no was the answer I wanted. (I recommend trying this with toddlers in the 'NO!' phase.) Do not worry, karma got me back. Now I have a head tremor!

Another way my mother showed me how to have fun with odd things was when she lost her eye. She suffered secondary glaucoma in her right eye and lost the sight. It was very painful so eventually she had her right eye removed. She of course got a fake eye. Unfortunately, the doctor tucked her eye lid the wrong way and so she went through a few eyes before they found one that worked, leaving her with extra eyes. One of the family stories was about a time when she and my father had gone to a fancy banquet in San Francisco for a Serra dinner. She was eating soup when all of a sudden she sneezed. She, being a lady, had gotten her napkin up in time. The lady next to her screamed!

My Mom looked down to see her eye floating in the soup. She spooned up her eye, and excused herself, and took it into the bathroom (presumably cleaned it off) before she put it back in, to remedy the situation. She put on an eye patch so it would not happen again. She laughed every time she told the story. I am sure she was embarrassed and she felt bad for the lady sitting next to her, but it was always good for a laugh at any family gathering. She always liked to add that later when she went outside for a smoke, someone put a quarter in her coffee cup because they thought she was pan-handling! Talk about adding insult to injury.

Do not feel sorry for her, she would not have wanted it. That is why one day when I came home from school, I found one of her eyes taped to the television. She was so proud when she told my brother and I that it was there to keep an eye on what we watched! She also told me I had to promise to behave on my first official date with a boy in high school. Otherwise, she said, I would have to take her eye on my date so . . . you guessed it, she could keep an eye on me. I was mortified as any early teen would be, but now I laugh at the memory.

I have Mom's eyes now. She gave me one of her extras and then I inherited another when she passed away in 2006. They continue to bring laughs. One was taped to a co-worker's computer monitor for almost a year because I taped it there as a joke and he loved it so much it stayed (until we had a client visit and his manager asked him to remove it!) I taped one to my refrigerator while I was losing weight.

2013

2013 was a pivotal year for me and a great illustration of how wholeness can unfold. It was a year of change. It can be easy for me to look at what has not been accomplished. How far there is still to go. It is so important for me to focus on the celebrations! I left my job at InsideTrack after almost five years. These years showed me that I could still contribute. I needed my work life to be different if I was going to have more vitality and thrive. I needed to work less and have more flexibility. I had discovered that I needed to start no earlier than 10 A.M. so that I did not have a huge dive in energy in the afternoon. I wanted more than setting work as a priority and having to settle for what was left-over for the rest of my life. I wanted more.

I developed my own coaching business that combines my gifts and allows me to be flexible. I can wake when it is best for my bio-rhythms and set appointments with recovery time between. I went to a wonderful conference in San Diego where I solidified the niche of working with people who live with chronic pain. Avita, a business consulting firm, was hired by Vocational Rehabilitation to conduct a business feasibility study and write a business plan with me. I got approved for start-up costs from Vocational Rehabilitation which included getting a great website designed.

I worked with five clients and impacted their lives positively. People from around the world visited my website and Facebook page. I designed the "Five Steps from Ow to Wow!" I launched the business with a party, interviewed practitioners, and did six radio show broadcasts. It was a year of stepping out, investing in myself, and developing the model that I use with clients. It was also scary. I could have stayed and tried to make it work at my job but I wanted to use my butterfly wings.

What Are You Thinking?

Affirmations, positive thoughts and attitudes are incredibly important to good health. Studies abound. The issue here is that it is easier said than done when your body is in pain. Everyone around you says that the pain would be better if you would just change your thinking. This is a lot like saying you just have to learn to live with it! How?!?!?!

ACT (Acceptance and Commitment Therapy) and CBT (Cognitive Behavioral Therapy) are two Psychological approaches to chronic pain that have been researched and shown to be helpful. One of the things that they both focus on are thoughts. If your thought patterns are mostly negative and defeating, this has an impact on your motivation; your behaviors; your bothersome response to pain; and your level of pain. If your thought patterns are mostly positive and hopeful this can have a positive impact on the same things. Mindfulness can help you to notice your thoughts. Noticing pulls you out of the reflex/react mode and allows a slight pause in which you can discover choice, which is when you can impact neuroplasticity and change patterns.

I consider myself an optimistic-depressive. The core of my beliefs is that life is good, that people are basically good, and that the world has beauty and purpose. Yet I have a propensity for depression in my genes. I was depressed as an adolescent and I have been diagnosed with bi-polar II which is a soft bi-polar. This diagnosis came after the accident. I now call depression 'the rabbit hole'. When I was in my teens it was 'the black hole'. The difference is that the black hole sucked me in whereas the rabbit hole entices me in, if I get too close.

I have learned over the years how to stay out of the rabbit hole but occasionally I go in, especially when I have more pain or it is around my period. Hormones play a role for me. To stay away from the rabbit hole, I focus on the positive—look at something beautiful, breathe, pet my dogs, list gratitudes, read a good book, color, walk, swim, eat good food, call a friend, visit nature, watch silly videos on the internet, read a favorite book, watch a heart-warming movie on television, or go to a movie. When the rabbit hole starts to entice, I deny it. No, I do have friends. No, it will not always be like this. No, I am loveable. No, I have something to contribute. No, I do have worth. No, I can breathe. These no's support my yes. My yes to life.

Mindfulness helps to uncover your default thinking. Where do your thoughts tend to go? Do you tend to think the very worst possible outcomes will happen (catastrophizing)? Our minds tend to go through the same worn paths. Just like the deer in the field wear down a path and then others follow, our thoughts tend to follow the same neuro-pathways. In order to change those paths, you must first become aware of your thinking so you can find new paths to forge.

Wishing and Hoping

Wishing, wanting, or demanding something that is not true right now is frustrating. Frustration can trigger the sympathetic nervous system—fight, flight, freeze. Your system goes on high alert; your muscles tense, your blood pressure increases, and your body does not absorb nutrients effectively. Living with chronic pain is exhausting. Wishing and hoping that things were different makes more fatigue and does not get you what you want. This way of being is the opposite of acceptance and mindfulness—it is rejecting the present, the gift of today.

Sure, I would prefer not to experience chronic pain. I would prefer to not get migraines. I would prefer to be able to eat whatever I want and not have to deal with weight gain or health issues. But accepting that these are things that I live with, lightens my load. I have more energy because I am not fighting what is. I can focus on my preferences and desires and create change one action at a time. Instead of refusing to accept, I empower myself to take action.

Being aware of your thoughts and emotions increases your ability to pause which allows you to make a choice which can engage your neuro-plasticity. This can impact your experience of pain. If something can be changed, it takes courage to take action. Action outside of yourself and within. Action takes hope that something can be affected-otherwise, why bother? Being present and positive, taking effective actions which are aligned with your values is what acceptance gives you; the power to take action and thrive.

If something cannot be changed, it is more powerful and life affirming to accept it in the moment and focus on what can be changed. I may not be able to be 50 pounds lighter right now, but I can love my body as it is and treat it well. The pounds are lost through my actions which are supported by my emotions and thoughts. It is also important to remember that does not mean that you stop because someone else tells you something is impossible. I met a man who had broken his neck and was told he would probably never walk again much less be able to play drums. (Unlike me, he actually was a drummer before the injury.) Now not only is he walking, he is in a band playing the drums, "better than before". He did not accept that he would never walk again. But neither did he wallow in the wishing and wanting it to be different. He put in the long, painful hours of physical therapy to make it different and to prove them wrong. He knew that their statistics did not mean him. He was an expert on himself and he used their words as motivation to act.

Bringing it all together

- No one else can know how you experience pain.
- You cannot do it alone but neither can anyone do it for you.
- Chronic pain and the treatment of it is complex.
- Turning have-to into get-to is an attitude adjustment that turns surviving into thriving.
- Living a life of Wow happens when you are willing to observe wonder!

- Going from Ow to Wow is both an inside job as well as an external job.
- Pain is a biological, psychological, and social phenomenon.
- Purpose creates meaning when you go beyond yourself.
- Meditation and mindfulness open you to the place where you can recognize wholeness.
- Actions, thoughts and emotions can co-create the ground of your experience.
- Support makes life worth living.
- You can be a Thriver and live a life of Wow!

If I truly want to be a concert pianist, I must do the work. In other words, act. I will never be a concert pianist because luckily for me, I do not really want to be a pianist! I am short three major ingredients. First, I do not know how to play the piano very well. Second, I have not put in the tens of thousands of hours of work. Third, I do not possess the desire that would allow me to acquire the first two. That does not stop me from imagining that I am the pianist in my tails at the grand piano when I am at a concert and the music washes over me. I may wish I could be that pianist in that moment, but it does not make it so.

If music is your passion, there are many ways to have it be a part of your life. Just because I will never be a concert pianist does not mean I cannot get a keyboard and teach myself. That is exactly what I did a few years ago. I grew up playing guitar and still do. In my late 20's, I got a saxophone and taught myself how to play. Again, I was not great and my roommate could tell you that *Strangers in the Night* can get really old, really quick! I still play keyboards and guitar for my own pleasure because I find it relaxing and fun. The wonder I experience with the music is part of my Wow!

In this last section of the book, we will explore how to create a Thriving with Pain Plan™. Written goals that include action steps and accountability have a significant more likelihood of success. If you truly want to move from Ow to Wow, I highly recommend that you take the time to find your leverage points and dive into the Five Steps from Ow to Wow by creating a plan, writing it down, include accountability and engage in powerful actions.

Exercise #18—Intention

Now that you have your core values, bring them into your everyday. When you wake each morning for at least three weeks, set an intention for your day of the type of experience you want to have. It can be joy, love, thrive, mindful . . . whatever fits for your values and you. Write it down. Then name one action you can do today to bring that intention into reality.

Exercise #19—Environment

Imagine how you feel when you are in an environment that is chaotic, loud, or with lots of stimulation that startles you. What does that feel like? Can you imagine a situation like that? Walk around this environment. Allow yourself to be fully present in this chaotic, loud, startling space. Be fully present and let the environment flow over you. What does your body feel like? What kind of emotional response do you have? Are you angry, frightened, or . . .? Are you relaxed or stressed? Do you notice any increase in pain levels? Now allow that witness part of you to come in and just notice, without judging your experience. What do you notice? As you feel your emotions without judging and you notice your thoughts without trying to correct them, do you notice anything shift?

Imagine how you feel when you are in an environment that feels peaceful, beautiful, or relaxing. What does that feel like? Can you imagine a situation like that? Walk around or sit in your mind's eye in this environment. What are the elements that you are imagining? What sounds, smells, sights, tastes, textures, temperature are you imagining for this place? Notice how your body feels. Are you relaxed or stressed? Do you notice any change in pain levels? Now allow that witness part of you to come in and just notice, without judging your experience. What do you notice? As you feel your emotions without judging and you notice your thoughts without trying to correct them, do you notice anything shift?

Exercise #20—Mindfulness

Take five breaths a day mindfully to begin your practice. Bring you attention to your breath. You do not need to change anything. Do not try to breath deeply, just bring your attention to the present and your breathing as it is. As you breathe in, say to yourself, "breathe in." As you breathe out, say to yourself, "breathe out."

As you feel confident that you are mindful with these breaths, you can add to your attending by following your breath all the way in and all the way out by saying in your mind, "I follow my breath all the way in, I follow my breath all the way out."

The next stage is to increase your awareness to part of your body as you breathe in and out and the final stage is to become aware of your whole body as you breathe in and out. As you widen your awareness to parts of your body as well as your whole body, remember that there is nothing to judge. You are being present with your experience and noticing.

Exercise #21—Laughter

What makes you laugh? If you can laugh at yourself, you have it made! Sometimes you may need a little help. Take the time to figure this out so that you can make sure to laugh at least once a day.

- Are there comics or comedians you enjoy?
- List a few of your favorite comedy movies.
- Find at least five *YouTube* channels that get you laughing.

Go to a movie with other people so you can catch the laughter.

Pets can be a great source of laughter. My dog, Pippin, is almost always a hit when we sit in the living room and he goes into the den and brings his bed out. It is bigger than him and he grabs it with his mouth and drags it in. It gets me every time!

Try Laughter Yoga.

Your Thriving with Pain Plan™

We have looked at the Five Steps and now it is time to use this information to transform your life from Ow to Wow. In other words, time for the rubber to hit the road. You will use the five skills that we have explored: awareness, action, connection, purpose and mindfulness to move toward your Wow. Every journey starts with a first step and it helps to know where you want to go; what pitfalls, barriers and obstacles you may face along the way; what your assets are such as your gifts, tools and talents; what you have in your tool box; who you have on your team; and where you are starting from. Just as you are unique, your vision and your Thriving with Pain Plan™ (TWP Plan) will be unique. This is definitely not a one size fits all approach!

Your Vision—Destination

The first step is to begin to unveil your vision. Remember the story of fire-walking? You go from point A to point B. You stay present and you keep your eye on your destination. The best plans begin with the end in mind. Maybe you already know exactly what you want and where you want to be. That is great!

Take some time to express that in a concrete way so that you can see your destination clearly as you take the steps to get there. This can be in words or a collage or a picture or a statue or . . . let your imagination run wild.

Maybe you are more in the goo stage and are unsure of what this can look like. That is great too! It is time for you to let the core of you, your DNA, so to speak, come out and play. It is time for you to reveal your core. If you have not done the exercise of finding your DNA from Step Four, do one of those and then come back here and create the concrete vision piece from above.

Maybe you know what you want but cannot imagine that you will ever get there. There is one sure way to never get there; not take the first step. It may be a bit of a leap of faith right now but I believe that our desires and yearnings hold within them a way to be manifested. Your destination may not look like you think it should but looking at what you want can reveal your core. This core may end up expressing differently than what you can imagine now or how you want it too, but it holds the seeds of your vision.

If you do not feel that you have any kind of vision at this time you may want to talk with a friend, meditate, write down your dreams, have a coaching session or go to counseling. You may be depressed and may need some support to see any light. As the light comes back, you can explore what you want. You can even use this exercise to help define the vision by choosing little things that spark joy, peace, or whatever values you hold high. Take at least one small action everyday.

Your vision can be grand which pulls you forward toward a shining destination or a smaller vision that reveals the next step. It does not matter. You are where you are right now and that is okay! Sometimes you are the caterpillar, sometimes the goo, sometimes the butterfly. One is not better than the other; when you accept what is, in the moment. By making something concrete that reflects and/or reveals your vision, you can keep your focus on your destination. My vision collages hang on my office wall to keep my focus on my thriving.

Here are a few ideas of how to make a concrete representation of your vision.

- Create an image collage of your vision
  - ◊ Create a collage by using old magazines and/or photos. This can be a fun creative project that can be done in stages so let's break it down.
    - * Find images that reflect what you want and create a visual depiction.
    - * Gather your supplies: scissors, glue stick, poster board (size of your choosing)—I usually recommend at least 8 ½ by 11in. You can add in glitter, stickers, or whatever makes you smile. (Put these altogether.)
    - * If you do not have these supplies, put them on your shopping list and pick them up as you are able. Ask a friend or two if they would like to join you and see if they can help gather supplies.
    - * Gather pictures that represent to you what you would like to create in your life. Some people like to tear pictures out in the evening when they are watching television or you may want to cut them out neatly. You do not need to know what each image represents, let your super and subconscious in to play. (As you gather the images, put them in a file with the other supplies.)
    - * Now it is time to assemble it. You can do this a little at a time if you find that it is too much to do in one sitting. Take your time and do not rush

it. It is your vision so it does not have to mean anything to anyone else. This is for you.

◊   Do the above and add words.
◊   Do the above but use online tools to gather images and/or words and put together in a collage or file that you can access easily. *www.ribbet.com/create-collage* and *www.smilebox.com/collages* are two options.

- If you paint, paint a picture. I once had a client who painted a picture that represented to her much of what she wanted and found it inspirational to look at.
- Get creative and use what you already do to represent your vision.
- Write a vision statement.
- Write a story that illustrates a day in your vision life.
- Write a slogan!

As you move forward with creating and implementing your TWP Plan, this becomes something that you can look at to keep you motivated and focused on your destination, your point B.

If you feel stuck or would like some inspiration, here are some questions to explore in meditation and/or in a journal.

- What do you want your life to look like, be like, and feel like?
- How do you want to feel and what do you think will help you get there?
- Where are you on this journey from Ow to Wow?
- What does 'Willingly Observing Wonder' mean to you in your life?

Within your vision are the seeds to your life of Wow and the fuel to make it a reality. Remember, you are moving toward your Wow. You are adding the "W" to the Ow through your willingness to observe wonder; recognizing wholeness; effective actions; building and sustaining connections; and living with purpose. Your TWP Plan supports you to not move away from Ow but rather toward your Wow!

Leverage Points

Creating a plan that holds the biggest bang for the buck can be a bit tricky. Pain is complex and it can be easy to feel that you need to change everything all at once. Now you have a vision, just get to it, right? Pain as well as fatigue and exhaustion may be barriers so you need to move forward smarter, not harder. The trick is finding goals that make a difference, are doable and will get you closer to your vision. You may already know what you want to do, what your first goal is. Great! Let us take that and lay it out and see how it lines up against the Steps. One goal can cover anywhere from one to all Five Steps.

Look at my example and then try it with your goal(s). If you do not have one, just check out the example for now. I mentioned in Step Three, the summer of 2014 I made a goal to work toward hiking in nature. A good plan begins with the end in mind. I had a vision; the vision of doing the Cascade Head hike by August in a way that did not exhaust me or increase pain. This goal utilized all Five Steps.

1. You are the Expert on You: Track progress—changes in fatigue, pain levels and use a FitBit to track steps.

Practice the skill of awareness through pacing, tracking tools and notice progress.

2. Use Your Treatment and Pain Management Options: Increase movement, exercise and healthy eating habits to manage pain.
3. Practice the skill of action through walking, stretching and eating habits.
4. Build Your Community: Hike and walk with friends. Practice the skill of connection through contact and communication around pacing.
5. Engage Your Passions, Purpose and Life: Being in nature is a huge value of mine.
6. Practice the skill of intention through remembering the meaning behind being in nature. (I got to be out in it a lot!)
7. Live Mindfully and Thrive: Be mindful and accept what is true in the moment.
8. Practice the skill of mindfulness through pacing and observing the wonders of nature.

Hiking the Cascade Head Trail was the big goal but I also knew it would mean spending lots of time in nature which was a big motivation. To keep the destination, the goal, in front of me, I put up a collage that included fresh vegetables, wonderful nature shots and walking trails. In order to reach a big goal, you need to figure out three things:

1. Where are you now? What is your point A? In April, when I began to work my Thriving with Pain Plan, I was in a flare up and could not walk to my nearby park without increasing my pain by at least 2 points. My muscles were deconditioned. I was eating healthy and had lost 50 pounds. This was my point A.

2. Where do you want to go? What is your point B (your destination)? By August I wanted to be able to hike the Cascade Head Trail without increasing pain and fatigue so that I could experience nature and friends.
3. What do you need in order to take the journey? I needed to take small steps to increase muscle conditioning and maintain flexibility. I also needed to observe wonder, honor my pace, obtain good walking shoes and hiking information, and walk with my community in order to stay motivated and be successful.

Once I knew what needed to be done, I needed a plan to get there. SMARTER goals are actionable goals that break down the big goal into bite size pieces. How big your bite is, is up to you. I find it more doable to break things down into smaller steps so I can pace myself and stay motivated. I also appreciate an inspiring goal, one I can feel enthusiastic about. First let us take a look at what SMARTER stands for. This is not an original concept. (Stephen Covey, for one, talks about this in his work.) Many people talk about SMART goals, but it can be useful to keep it in mind as you make your TWP Plan.

SMARTER stands for:

S – Specific: concrete and specific not vague

M – Measureable: able to check off a list because you know it is completed

A – Accountable: have ways to stay on track and motivated

R – Realistic: be realistic about what can be done

T – Timeline: have timeframes so it is not done "someday"

E – Enthusiastic: make it something you can get excited about

R – Rewarding: have a clear reward for accomplishing goal

My TWP Plan included re-establishing good pacing in order to get back in condition by listening to my body. Since I hike with friends, I needed to be willing to take care of myself, have a way to communicate and take the time I needed to rest in order to set a comfortable but challenging pace. I needed to start slowly, keep going and increase the difficulties of walks and hikes throughout the summer. This allowed me to increase my stamina and get my legs in better shape, while taking care of my lower back. I had to take days off from walking after hikes to let my body heal. I needed to balance action, rest, and motivation. Following is my TWP Plan for this vision.

Goal	Specific	Measure	Account-able	Realistic	Time Bound	Enthusiastic Reward
Eat Healthy Eat 5 veggie servings, no sugar and no dairy	X 5-6 meals a day. Take multi-vitamins	X Keep food log everyday	X Do with partner. Food Log, weigh once a week	X Yes, we are both on plan and treats are out of the house	X 2 months	X Feel better & lighter.
Walk daily. Slowly increase distance.	X Start with walking around block and add 10% per week	X Use Fitbit to track length of walks	X Go with Rhiannon and put on calendar	X Most of the time. Need to pace and be gentle when needed.	X Walk at least once a day.	X Watch a favorite show after the walk or make popcorn.
One hike per week. Increase difficulty	X Take a hike each weekend	X Schedule	X Make dates with friends & pick hikes	X I have time, honor pacing	X Slow increase	X Being in nature!
Stretch routine for lower body in am and upper body pm	X	X Create tracking sheet and put it up	X Tracking visible for me & partner	X Yes, gentle so able to do most days	X Do for 2 months	X Some thing fun Dog snuggle or coloring time.

I walked almost every day around my neighborhood, stretched to increase flexibility and continued to eat healthy. All of this took action steps. I had to be motivated, to believe that it was possible and to take action. I also had to be patient. There were days I could not walk or didn't follow through. The day after challenging hikes, I was so exhausted that I did not do any walking. I had a lot of support from my friends emotionally, physically and mentally. They helped me to stay motivated, set up dates for the hiking, figured out walks and hikes that fit my abilities and went at my pace. The dates helped to hold me accountable which was important on a weekend when my motivation might be low. Action buddies are a great way to stay motivated, be accountable and go beyond yourself. Who wants to let your friends down? It was important that I did not overdo it though.

I could have easily hung out in Ow by not allowing myself to even dream of the possibility that I could do an eight mile, 1000-foot elevation change hike. The reality in April supported that assessment. Instead I followed my Wow. I decided on a destination to aspire to. I created a concrete visual depiction to inspire and motivate me. I made sure that the path included the elements of the destination that I wanted; community, mindfulness and time outside in nature. One day, one step at a time I went from A to B. I spent most weekends taking one hike with friends. I spent most days being kind to myself with good eating habits, pacing around walking and gentle stretching. I created a plan that was easy to follow and had all the elements of SMARTER goals and all of the Five Steps. I followed through with some help from my friends. I did get to do the Cascade Head Trail. The beauty of this plan was that even if I did not make the final goal, I got everything I wanted along the way; time in nature, pain management and time with friends! I got there by keeping my eye on the destination and focusing on one thing at a time.

Create your plan

What does a life of Wow look like to you right now? What can you imagine as your destination? In my example, I saw being with friends, hiking and being out in nature as an important destination. It fed my soul. What is important to you right now? Take the time right now to write it down.

My vision of my Wow:

What is your big goal that will help you move toward your Wow?

Mark below the Steps that you see are part of this goal:

Step One: You are the Expert on You   Skill of Awareness

Step Two: Know Your Treatment Options   Skill of Action

Step Three: Build Your Community   Skill of Connection

Step Four: Engage Your Passions   Skill of Intention

Step Five: Live Mindfully and Thrive   Skill of Mindfulness

What other big goal will help you move toward your Wow?

Mark below the Steps that you see are part of this goal:

Step One: You are the Expert on You   Skill of Awareness

Step Two: Know Your Treatment Options   Skill of Action

Step Three: Build Your Community   Skill of Connection

Step Four: Engage Your Passions   Skill of Intention

Step Five: Live Mindfully and Thrive   Skill of Mindfulness

What other big goal will help you move toward your Wow?

Mark below the Steps that you see are part of this goal:

Step One: You are the Expert on You   Skill of Awareness

Step Two: Know Your Treatment Options   Skill of Action

Step Three: Build Your Community   Skill of Connection

Step Four: Engage Your Passions   Skill of Intention

Step Five: Live Mindfully and Thrive   Skill of Mindfulness

Take a look at these big goals that you wrote and your vision of your Wow. Do you feel inspired? Do you believe that it is possible to reach these goals? If the answer to these questions is YES, then it is time to build a plan. If the answer to these questions is no or maybe, how can you change them so the answer is YES? To live a life of Wow you need inspiring goals that you believe in, ones that support you to thrive. Your belief does not have to be 100% all the time. As a matter of fact, it is better if your goals stretch you. When I set the goal of hiking the Cascade Head, it was not a "but of course" goal. It was a stretch. I knew there was work that I needed to do. I knew there was a possibility that I would not be able to reach the goal since my back was flaring up. The goal was inspiring because it was something I really wanted and I knew it would help me with all Five Steps. It gave me a big bang for my buck. The reward of taking those hikes made all of the daily walking, eating well, and stretching well worth it and I was in better shape so I felt better.

Now choose one goal, one destination for your Thriving with Pain Plan™. Enthusiasm can be dangerous to those of us who live with chronic pain. You can make a decision and find yourself doing great for a while. You may make some great progress and then, SPLAT. You end up in so much pain that the whole experience becomes one more thing that you never want to do again because you have overwhelmed yourself. I had a dream that illustrates why it is so important to focus on one thing at a time. In the dream, I found myself at my childhood home trying to get to the front door to get in. The house was on a hill and I found myself on a very steep driveway. This made no sense since my parents are dead and they never lived on a hill. Nonetheless, here I was trying to get up an incredibly steep driveway to the garage. I struggled up three-quarters of the way and then slipped back down. I tried again. Exhausted, I slipped down to the bottom of the driveway. I was incredulous. How did my 80-year-old mother get up there? I found myself getting angry, she shouldn't live up here by herself! Then I saw her come down the street and she turned into a walkway that had stairs that took her to the front door. She went up them without any struggle. Duh! It is not the distance or steepness; it is the way you go about it that makes the difference. I was fighting gravity on a slick, steep surface. My mother took the stairs one at a time. Each step gives a moment of stability, a place to rest if needed. You don't need to struggle up the hill all at once, if you try, you slide back down and end up at the beginning again or worse, SPLAT!

It does not matter what you choose to start with as long as it is something that will bring you closer to your vision of a life of Wow. It can be small and may seem mundane but if it inspires you, that is what is important. Maybe it is as simple as finding the one place in your house for your keys and your purse or wallet. Getting into the habit of putting it there reduces stress when you go to look for it. This is a proactive strategy!

Once you have decided on your one big goal it is time to create the plan.

- What do you need in order to make this goal happen? (This can be anything from support, time, motivation, information, or materials.)
- What action steps? (What can you do to move toward this goal? Eat right vs lose weight.)
- Who do you need on your team? (Pick your team and ask if they are available.)
- What kind of tracking or awareness do you need to bring so that you can stay on track and be effective?

Fill in the Plan below or go to *www.thrivingwithpain.com* to download more blanks. Make sure that the goals are actionable which means you have some influence over whether or not it happens; they are specific and not vague; they are measurable and realistic for you right now; you have some accountability; they are time bound; and, you have enthusiasm and a reward connected to your accomplishing it.

Thriving with Pain Plan™

Goal	Specific	Measure	Accountable	Realistic	Time Bound	Enthusiasti Reward

An example of a non-actionable goal is losing weight. An actionable goal that could help you to achieve weight loss may be eating a certain number of vegetable servings or calories or portion size. You can do that and know it has been done but putting the goal on something that you may not be able to predict is disempowering. Focus on what you can do and not the end result. I know this seems contradictory to the idea of a destination and a big vision. The vision helps you to want to take the steps and the steps move you toward the vision. You can meditate everyday and have the vision be feeling less stress and more peaceful. Meditating is within your influence because it is an action you can take. You cannot 'do' less stress but you can practice stress management. Un-actionable goals set you up for frustration. Work within what you can influence. It is like someone telling you to relax. I'm trying! How relaxing is that? Not very. But if you were to do deep diaphragmatic breathing, you might relax.

Putting Together a Breakthrough Pain Plan

One plan that everyone who lives with chronic pain needs is a pain management/coping plan, especially for break-through pain. When you live with pain it can be difficult to remember what to do when a new wave hits. All of the muscle/nerve memory of past pain seems to be triggered and it is easy to forget what to do. That is why a plan that you can refer to is so important. What helps you to remember?

You can develop a kit that has reminders of your tools and actual tools. You may want to have it clearly marked for a particular kind of pain such as a migraine or lower back flare. What are your tools? For migraines, I have a box with three Maxalt (which is the maximum I can take in 24 hours), an essential oil blend, a card that says "ice pack on your neck—in the freezer", a card that says "warm footbath with Epsom salts and essential oil", a card that says "go to bed, close your eyes, put the blanket over your head!", nasal spray, a card that says "pressure points between thumb and index finger, bridge of nose, and base of occiput", a card that says "passive sensory attention of feet on mp3 player", a card that says "autogenic cooling blue glow on mp3 player" and a card that says "cookie in fridge" for a cannabis cookie when I have nothing I need to do for the rest of the day (I live in a state where that is legal). Obviously I have a lot of tools in my tool box but I did not start with that. You can start with what you have now and add as you find things that support you. Having it all in one place reduces the "trying to figure it out" when you are not feeling well. You can also add your support people to reach out to. Your toolbox is to assist you in doing what you know you can do—if you could only remember to!

Every day is an opportunity to make a choice. Are you going to thrive or are you going to let go of your power? Sometimes this takes the form of being gentle and allowing yourself to rest. You may want to do one gentle visualization or meditation that supports you in recovering, pain management and/or soothing your Sympathetic Nervous System. Remember it is about how you live that creates thriving and your Wow. It is not about you struggling or fighting against. It is not always easy. Sometimes you have to push beyond what you feel like doing in the moment and act. Sometimes you have to rest when you feel restless and want to act. Both can be true. It is a delicate dance of balance. With your willingness you can observe wonder, develop the skills to manage pain, discover motivations, create new habits, and live a thriving life. It usually does not happen over night. Slowly, with perseverance and actions, you can find your own way to thrive.

How the Steps Fit into Your Plan

When you build your Thriving with Pain Plan™, make it inspiring: be realistic, stretch yourself and do not overdo it. Each Step and skill fits into a strong and inspiring Plan. Willingly observe wonder as you envision and move toward your vision of a thriving life. Use the skills of self-awareness/stalking, action, community, purpose, and mindfulness to move toward more Wow! Once you have set out a plan, look at it to make sure that it takes into account all of the aspects of Thriving with Pain.

Let's begin with Step One so that you get to know what is a realistic stretch goals. You may already know that you tend to over-do it, so you want to make sure that you do not stretch yourself too much. Or you may know that you tend to not stretch yourself enough, so you want to make sure you are really creating stretch goals. What can you do to increase your own expertise? Self-stalking! Be honest about yourself and your tendencies. Being an expert on yourself supports movement toward a more effective Thriving with Pain Plan™. You can adjust your plan as you discover more about what works and what does not work for you. The Plan is there to serve you, not the other way around. **Make sure that tracking is included**.

Step Two's skill is action which is required to live your Wow. You do not necessarily have to set out actions that are a big struggle to accomplish. Instead, they can be small and quiet such as listening to music, reading inspiring or entertaining material, doing a visualization, phoning a friend, deep breathing, or even following through with your treatment plans. As you look at your TWP Plan what action(s) can you take daily that move you toward your vision and/or will interrupt the cycle of pain and engage the Thriving Cycle? **Make sure that the goals within your TWP Plan are actionable**.

Step Three is all about building your community. Remember that you are not alone. Hundreds of millions of people live with chronic pain and many suffer in silence. Many people tend to not be open about their pain because of the stigma. How does your TWP Plan support you to erase the barriers, overcome isolation and connect with your community? Just because you cannot do the things you used to, does not mean you cannot connect. Your presence, a phone call, an email, a handwritten note or a card maybe what is needed to bridge the isolation and connect. Who can you connect with today to build and sustain your community?

Step Four is where thriving comes into full view. Purpose, passion, and meaning are the fuel for aliveness and support you to move beyond survival. As you move toward your purpose, passion, and engage meaning in your life, your goals and vision inspire you to thrive. By developing your skill of intention, you are able to live in an empowered place of choice. How is your intention reflected in your TWP Plan? To live on purpose everyday, finish this sentence; I am a thriver today because . . . Or ask yourself, "Why am I such a great thriver?"

Living mindfully and thriving is what Step Five is all about. When you are told to just learn to accept it, this step is how you do that. After you engage your courage and wisdom, you can find that place of acceptance where you can activate the skill of mindfulness. Living your Wow is an ongoing process that is an empowered acceptance in each moment. How does your plan include mindful thriving?

Wow takes willingness to accept and act. It is not always easy to discern what is needed in each moment. When in doubt, go to the steps and skills from the Ow to Wow model. These questions can assist you to discern what might be a good place to focus.

- Are you in alignment with what you know is true for you?
- Is there something you can do to improve your situation?
- Can you connect with others to lessen isolation?
- What is your intention?
- Are you fully present in this moment?

I have moments and sometimes a whole day that I allow myself to wallow in the 'what if' and the 'if only'. Wallowing or inviting in the angry part of me can help to shake things up but if I allow it to take over, it gets in the way of thriving. When I bemoan that things are not the way they were before, I am in denial and out of acceptance. I am not sure things were ever the way that part of me remembers. I am human. So I do not beat myself up when this happens. The anger and self-pity block expression of what is true now. Instead, the focus is on anything rather than accepting what is. This is exhausting and fruitless. When I remember that as long as there is life, there is purpose, I am able to re-align with my values and purpose.

When I accept what is in the moment, the experience of acceptance turns on my Parasympathetic Nervous System and allows me to relax into the present moment of 'now'. This allows me to live in flow instead of resistance and turns down the volume of my experience of pain. Willingly observing wonder creates your WOW. Go forth and THRIVE!

---

[i]On Grief and Grieving: Finding the Meaning of Grief Through the Five Stages of Loss Elisabeth Kubler Ross
[ii]www.dominican.edu/academics/ahss/undergraduate-programs/psych/faculty/assets-gail-matthews/researchsummary2.pdf

Author Biography

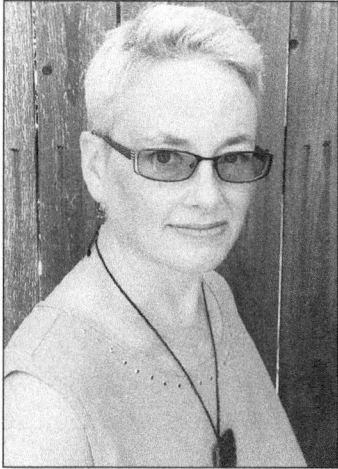

Amber Rose Dullea, MA, M.Div. is an inspiring coach, speaker and author. She brings an embodied compassion to her work due to living for over a decade with Fibromyalgia and chronic migraines. She combines compassion and humor with her background as a Licensed Massage Therapist. Her nurturing coaching skills support individuals who live with chronic pain to thrive again by finding and living their Wow!

Amber Rose earned her Master's Degree in Whole Systems Design with a focus on Personal and Planetary Healing from Antioch University in Seattle, Master of Divinity in Interfaith and New Thought from New West Seminary, and a B.A. Special Major in Peace and Conflict Studies. She has served as faculty at Marylhurst University, Oregon School of Massage, Renton Community College and serves as Secretary on the Mastering Pain Institute, Portland Progressive Toastmasters Boards of Directors, and is a public member on the Oregon Pain Management Commission.

Founder of Thriving with Pain LLC

Contact Information
* Website: www.thrivingwithpain.com
* Email: amberrose@thrivingwithpain.com
* Phone: 503-810-4163

Available Services

One-on-one Thriving with Pain Coaching
Engage with the Five Steps for Thriving with Pain with the assistance of a Coach who has been there. Design your Thriving with Pain Plan™, have support, short-cuts, and accountability to implement and live your WOW!
* **Certificate of Completion** from the *National Society of Health Coaches* in **Evidence-based Health Coaching**
* Coaching training through *InsideTrack Inc.* including Certified Master Coach, Coach Mentor, and Training in Career Coaching

Group Facilitation
Support groups, professional associations, Unity of Beaverton, Abundant Life Center and Non-profits

Motivational Speaker
Topics Include: Healthcare, Personal and Patient Empowerment, Compassionate Care
* "Living your Life of Wow!"—Florence Unitarian Universalist Fellowship **(Video Available)** www.youtube.com/watch?v=_1IfpiQaU2w
* "Making the Connections"—Abundant Life Center
* Conference and Symposium Presenter (Including Master

of Ceremony and Presenter at Antioch University, Seattle Whole Systems Design Symposium, "Diversity & Connections" and Presenter at Oregon Massage Therapy Association Conference)

- Advanced Communicator Bronze Award through Toastmasters International
- Winner Humorous Speech Club Contest (Portland Club), 2015

Workshops and Seminars

Topics Include: Thriving with Pain, Compassionate Care, Humor through Adversity, Whole Systems

- Oregon Vocational Rehabilitation Services, Antioch University, Seattle, Marylhurst University, Oregon School of Massage, Ashmead College
  - * Five Steps to Thriving with Pain, Aromatherapy, Massage Therapy, Ergonomics, Organizational Transformation, Systems Theory, Relationship with the Environment, Personal and Planetary Healing--Making the Connections, Change Theory, and Advanced Systems

Publications:

- *Pain Pathways Magazine*—*"Thriving—Ow to Wow!"*, Spring 2016 Issue
- *National Pain News*—"My Pain Story: Thriving with Pain" www.americannewsreport.com/nationalpainreport/my-story-thriving-with-pain-8820472.html
- Articles on www.thrivingwithpain.com
- Dullea, C. Amber Rose, *Path of Heart: Person and Planetary Healing*, 2002.
- Dullea, C. Amber Rose, *Making the Connections Person and Planetary Healing Workbook*, 1998.

www.ingramcontent.com/pod-product-compliance
Lightning Source LLC
Chambersburg PA
CBHW032136020426
42334CB00016B/1180